VACCINES

WHAT EVERYONE NEEDS TO KNOW®

VACCINES

WHAT EVERYONE NEEDS TO KNOW®

KRISTEN A. FEEMSTER

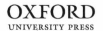
OXFORD

UNIVERSITY PRESS

OXFORD
UNIVERSITY PRESS

Oxford University Press is a department of the University of Oxford. It furthers
the University's objective of excellence in research, scholarship, and education
by publishing worldwide. Oxford is a registered trade mark of Oxford University
Press in the UK and certain other countries.

"What Everyone Needs to Know" is a registered trademark
of Oxford University Press.

Published in the United States of America by Oxford University Press
198 Madison Avenue, New York, NY 10016, United States of America.

Library of Congress Cataloging-in-Publication
Data Names: Feemster, Kristen A., author.
Title: Vaccines : what everyone needs to know / Kristen A. Feemster.
Description: New York, NY : Oxford University Press, [2017] |
Includes bibliographical references and index.
Identifiers: LCCN 2017033339 | ISBN 9780190277901
(hardcover : alk. paper) | ISBN 9780190277918 (paperback : alk. paper)
Subjects: LCSH: Vaccination—Popular works. |
Vaccination—History. | Vaccines.
Classification: LCC RA638 .F44 2017 |
DDC 614.4/7—dc23
LC record available at https://lccn.loc.gov/2017033339

This material is not intended to be, and should not be considered, a substitute for
medical or other professional advice. Treatment for the conditions described in this
material is highly dependent on the individual circumstances. And, while this material
is designed to offer accurate information with respect to the subject matter covered
and to be current as of the time it was written, research and knowledge about medical
and health issues is constantly evolving and dose schedules for medications are being
revised continually, with new side effects recognized and accounted for regularly.
Readers must therefore always check the product information and clinical procedures
with the most up-to-date published product information and data sheets provided by
the manufacturers and the most recent codes of conduct and safety regulation. The
publisher and the authors make no representations or warranties to readers, express
or implied, as to the accuracy or completeness of this material. Without limiting the
foregoing, the publisher and the authors make no representations or warranties as to
the accuracy or efficacy of the drug dosages mentioned in the material. The authors
and the publisher do not accept, and expressly disclaim, any responsibility for any
liability, loss or risk that may be claimed or incurred as a consequence of the use and/
or application of any of the contents of this material.

Hardback printed by Bridgeport National Bindery, Inc., United States of America

With love to James and our sunshines, TE and FM.
In memoriam to Mom, my greatest superhero.

CONTENTS

4. Vaccine Financing and Distribution   **51**

5. Vaccine Safety   69

7. Laws and Standard Practices for Vaccine Administration

8. Vaccine Hesitancy 125

9. On the Horizon   **139**

ACKNOWLEDGMENTS

Thank you: To Karen Smith, for your activation energy and for helping me find the right voice for this book. To my editor, CZ, for your patience and enthusiasm for this project. To my colleagues at the Children's Hospital of Philadelphia Division of Infectious Diseases and the Philadelphia Department of Public Health Immunization Program—I have learned from your insights, perspectives, and advocacy. To PolicyLab, for championing this important topic. To Bardia Nabet, Tunmise Fawole, and Charlotte Moser for help with figures and the appendix. To Paul Offit, for your critical feedback and guidance throughout. To my sister, Kara, for cheering me onward. And, most important, to my family for encouraging me to pursue this opportunity and for all of your support every step of the way.

ABBREVIATIONS

AAFP	American Academy of Family Physcians
AAP	American Academy of Pediatrics
ACCV	Advisory Commission on Childhood Vaccines
ACIP	Advisory Committee on Immunization Practices
ACOG	American College of Obstetricians and Gynecologists
ACP	American College of Physicians
BCG	Bacilli Calmette- Guérin
CDC	Centers for Disease Control and Prevention
CEP	Coalition for Epidemic Preparedness
CISA	Clinical Immunization Safety Assessment
DTaP	Diphtheria, Tetanus and acellular Pertussis vaccine
DTP	Diphtheria, Tetanus and whole cell Pertussis vaccine
EMA	European Medicines Agency
EPI	Expanded Program on Immunization
EU	European Union
FDA	Food and Drug Administration
GAVI	Global Alliance for Vaccines and Immunizations
GBS	Group B Streptococcus
GBS	Guillain–Barré syndrome
GCP	Guideline for Good Clinical Practice
HAV	Hepatitis A virus
HHS	Health and Human Services
HiB	Haemophilus influenza Type B
HIV	Human immunodeficiency virus

HPV	Human papillomavirus
ICH	International Conference on Harmonisation
IIV	Inactivated influenza vaccine
IND	Investigational New Drug
IOM	Institute of Medicine
IPV	Inactivated poliovirus vaccine
IVIG	Intravenous immunoglobulin
LAIV	Live attenuated influenza vaccine
MCV	Meningococcal conjugate vaccine
MMR	Measles, Mumps and Rubella vaccine
NAM	National Academy of Medicine
NIH	National Institutes of Health
NVAC	National Vaccine Advisory Committee
NVICP	National Vaccine Injury Compensation Program
NVPO	National Vaccine Program Office
PATH	Program for Appropriate Technology in Health
PCV	Pneumococcal conjugate vaccine
PRISM	Post-licensure rapid immunization safety monitoring
QALY	Quality-adjusted life year
RSV	Respiratory syncytial virus
SAGE	Strategic Advisory Group of Experts
SIRVA	Shoulder Injury Resulting from Vaccine Administration
Tdap	Tetanus, diphtheria and acellular pertussis vaccine
VAERS	Vaccine Adverse Events Reporting System
VFC	Vaccines for Children
VSD	Vaccine Safety Datalink
VZV	Varicella Zoster Vaccine
WHO	World Health Organization

INTRODUCTION

Vaccines represent one of the greatest public health advances of the past 100 years. Their development has brought about the global eradication of smallpox as well as large reductions in poliomyelitis, measles, tetanus, *Haemophilus influenzae* type b (Hib—a leading cause of childhood infections), and many other infectious diseases.

However, the development and implementation of vaccines has not followed a linear trajectory: Disparities in the adoption of new vaccines continue to persist, and vaccination rates in both developed and developing countries are not always sustained. These disparities may be attributable to short supply, poor infrastructure, or low prioritization of vaccines in public health spending. However, another important contributor to the success of vaccination programs is *vaccine acceptance*, a blanket term referring to the public cooperation with public vaccination schedules. As the perceived risk of vaccine-preventable diseases decreases, concerns about vaccine safety increase. This has contributed to a rise in vaccine hesitancy in many communities. Health care providers today spend considerable time and effort educating patients and families on the importance of immunization.

It has become difficult to identify resources that can adequately answer the public's questions about the risk and benefits of the ever-expanding list of vaccines available today. This is further complicated by the rapid proliferation and dissemination of misinformation from sources as varied as social media and scientifically unsound research articles. Recent outbreaks throughout the world show that vaccine-preventable diseases such as pertussis and measles can occur as vaccine hesitancy increases and immunization rates decrease. This highlights the importance of communication and trust between health care providers, patients, and the community to ensure the successful implementation of immunization programs. Many countries also continue to face challenges in ensuring reliable access to vaccines, which can further erode trust in the public health and medical system.

Vaccines are a public health tool: The decision to vaccinate or not vaccinate impacts both individuals and the people around them. Accordingly, it is imperative that we are well-informed before making a decision about vaccination. This requires an understanding of (1) how vaccines work, (2) the diseases that vaccines prevent, and (3) why vaccines are important for individuals and society. Vaccines and their role in society represent a complex interplay between sociopolitical systems, culture, economics, individual beliefs, and health literacy—and with that, they provide a multitude of fronts for the introduction of conflicting messages or incorrect information. This book aims to provide an objective, informative tool to communicate facts about vaccines as well as the challenges to implementing immunization on a population level.

1

WHAT IS A VACCINE AND HOW DO VACCINES WORK?

A vaccine is a substance that is given to a person or animal to protect it from a particular pathogen—a bacterium, virus, or other microorganism that can cause disease. The vaccine prompts an immune response in the body that produces antibodies, which are proteins that fight specific pathogens. The goal of giving a vaccine is to prompt the body to create antibodies specific to the particular pathogen, which in turn will prevent infection or disease; it mimics infection on a small scale that does not induce actual illness. A similar process does occur when the body confronts actual pathogens, but vaccines spare individuals from the dangers of disease.

A vaccine can be made from any one of a variety of sources: a killed or weakened bacteria or virus, a protein or sugar from the pathogen, or a synthetic substitute. For a vaccine to do its job, the following need to happen: (1) The vaccine needs to stimulate antibody production, and (2) the antibodies need to have avidity (attraction to the specific pathogen). Antibodies will not work if they do not bind to the invading pathogen. Vaccine protection also requires that the body recognize the pathogen and keep making antibodies when they are needed, which is called *immune memory*. When this happens, the vaccinated body is ready to produce more of these antibodies right away, whenever the body is exposed to the bacteria or virus.

What is an antigen?

Antigens are proteins on the surface of a pathogen that prompt the production of antibodies by the immune system. Bacteria and viruses are both covered in antigens, and during the process of natural infection, these antigens are what the body recognizes. Depending on the pathogen, its antigen coating can be made up of several proteins or several thousand.

Vaccines, on the other hand, are often made using just a few antigens from a bacteria or virus. This is because some antigens are better than others at sparking the immune system. This is also because it is important to separate the parts of a pathogen that cause disease and make one sick from those that induce an antibody response. The ability to cause disease is called *virulence*, whereas the ability to induce a protective immune response is called *immunogenicity*.

The number of antigens in vaccines is actually quite small compared to the number of antigens that confront the immune system during an actual infection (or just from the environment on a daily basis). For example, the pathogen that causes whooping cough contains more than 3,000 antigens; the vaccine that is used to protect against whooping cough contains only 3–5 different antigens. Our immune systems are stimulated all the time, but all stimulation is not the same.

What happens when the immune system is confronted by an antigen?

When one's body encounters an antigen (from either a vaccine or a natural exposure), it sparks a cascade of events that constitute an immune response. This response requires communication between several different types of cells and ends in the creation of *memory cells* that are equipped to respond to future invasions by the same antigen. When antigens are introduced as part of a vaccine, the steps essentially are as follows:

1. Antigen is picked up by an *antigen-presenting cell* that shows the antigen to a type of immune cell called a *helper T cell.*
2. Helper T cells activate *B cells* (these make antibodies) or *killer T cells* (needed to attack pathogens such as viruses that live inside of cells).
3. The activated B cells and killer T cells become *memory immune cells* that will reactivate during actual infection and keep the pathogen from invading.

How do cells signal each other in the process of creating antibodies?

Immune cells emit signals through the secretion of *cytokines.* Cytokines are crucial to our immune response in that they recruit all the cells we need to attack antigens and create memory cells. Some cytokines are also responsible for the symptoms that are generally associated with infection, such as fever. This is why we may experience a low fever after vaccination: It means our immune system is in the process of making memory cells, and cytokines are being employed as part of the communication between cells that contributes to this process.

Which is better, natural immunity or immunity after vaccination?

In general, natural infection results in a more robust, durable immune response. This is because an actual infection usually results in a stronger immune response (not to mention an actual illness), whereas we may need more than one dose of a vaccine to achieve full protective immunity. After infection, we make a greater number and greater diversity of antibodies—ones that may recognize different parts of a pathogen (i.e., its antigens). In the case of some pathogens, such as chickenpox and measles, infection results in lifelong immunity.

However, this is not the case for all pathogens. For example, immunity decreases over time after a pertussis (whooping cough) infection. Children younger than age 2 years who are infected with a certain family of bacteria are not able to mount an immune response that makes memory cells, so even after infection, they have no long-lasting immunity. If a virus or bacteria has multiple strains, infection with one strain may not provide immunity against other strains.

Some vaccines induce a stronger immune response than natural infection. One example is the human papillomavirus (HPV) vaccines, which are made from a purified capsid protein that induces higher antibody levels than are seen in individuals who have had actual HPV infection. The same is true of tetanus vaccines: Those who receive the vaccine have more antibodies than those who survive infection.

However natural immunity may compare to vaccine immunity for a given disease, it is important to remember that natural immunity comes with the cost of having to endure a disease or infection, which depending on the illness can result in disability or death.

What is the real risk of vaccine-preventable diseases?

Since the advent of vaccines, the incidence of vaccine-preventable diseases has decreased dramatically. The risk of being exposed to many of these diseases is therefore quite low, and some diseases (including polio and diphtheria) have been eliminated from the United States. For other vaccine-preventable disease, overall incidence has decreased but cases still occur because available vaccines do not cover all of the different types of the bacteria or virus. For example, the bacterium *Pneumococcus*, for which a vaccine has existed since the 1980s, continues to cause tens of thousands of cases of pneumonia, bloodstream infections, and meningitis every year.

On the other hand, the incidence of some vaccine-preventable diseases has persisted and even increased in recent years. Pertussis (whooping cough) cases have increased steadily since the 1980s, with nearly 50,000 cases reported in the United States in 2012. Pertussis affects all age groups, although infants have the highest risk of severe disease and typically require hospitalization. There are also regular outbreaks of vaccine-preventable diseases such as mumps, varicella, measles, and *Meningococcus* (which causes bloodstream infections and meningitis) in the United States and internationally. In places where there is reliable access to a developed medical system, the risk of death due to infection with any of these pathogens is low, but severe disease can and does still occur. The global risk of death due to pertussis among infected infants is approximately 1 in 100; for measles it is 1 in 1,000; and for *Meningococcus* across all age groups, the fatality rate for infected individuals is 1 in 10.

Thus, the actual risk of contracting a vaccine-preventable disease is difficult to project. Outbreaks of vaccine-preventable diseases generally occur when there are clusters of susceptible individuals or people who do not have immunity. When this happens, there is nothing to stop the virus or bacteria from moving between people. This is a larger issue for pathogens that are easily spread from person to person, such as pertussis or measles. Vaccination works by reducing the number of susceptible individuals, thereby stopping transmission; the bacteria or virus simply runs out of places to go. This is called *herd immunity*.

What is herd immunity?

Vaccines work by protecting the individual who is vaccinated. A vaccinated individual is less likely to become infected, and if the individual is not infected, he or she cannot spread the infection to others. When there are many vaccinated people in a community, there is nowhere for the bacteria or virus to go—the group, or herd, becomes immune. So even if there are a few individuals who are not vaccinated in the group, they are protected because there is no one around to expose them to the infection. This works better for some infections compared to others. Viruses or bacteria that are easily transmitted, including measles and pertussis (whooping cough), require that almost everyone in a given group be vaccinated in order to achieve herd immunity. Other infections require close contact for longer periods of time in order for exposure to result in infection. In these cases, a lower immunization rate can achieve herd immunity. In this manner, vaccines have had greater impact on disease rates than they would if every disease required uniform vaccination rates.

What happens when immunization rates are not high enough to achieve herd immunity?

When immunization rates are low, more individuals are susceptible to infection and are at risk of becoming infected. If anyone does become infected, the lower the immunization rate, the more opportunities there will be to spread the infection to other susceptible individuals in their group. When several cases such as this cluster together, an outbreak occurs. Outbreaks grow as long as there are more susceptible people in a given community to become infected and expose others. Outbreaks slow and eventually end when enough people are immune—either because of infection or because of vaccination.

How large are most outbreaks?

The size of an outbreak depends on the number of susceptible people, the infectivity (or contagiousness) of the pathogen, and the severity of disease caused by infection. For example, if a pathogen causes people to become very sick very quickly, there may be less opportunity for those individuals to go out and infect others. However, some pathogens, such as pertussis, can be transmitted before people even know they are infected, making these infections more difficult to control once they have started spreading in a community. This is why vaccines are used as a response to outbreaks: They prevent people from becoming infected in the first place.

What is the difference between immunization and vaccination?

Immunization refers to any exposure that provides immunity, which means that it encompasses both vaccination and natural infection. Immunization is often referred to as *active* or *passive*. Active immunization occurs when an individual is exposed to an antigen and then has an immune response that produces antibodies. Thus, active immunization can take place through vaccination or natural infection.

Passive immunization occurs when an individual receives antibodies from other than a first-hand immune response. The most common form of passive immunity is pregnant mothers passing antibodies to their fetuses through the placenta; this provides immune protection to infants for the first several months of their lives. Another form of passive immunization occurs through medical intervention, particularly for people with immunodeficiencies that keep them from making their own antibodies. In these cases, the immunodeficient individual may receive a blood product that contains antibodies pooled from other people. In cases of exposures to certain infections, including rabies, a person may be injected with a set of rabies-specific antibodies to provide immediate protection. These antibodies are short-lived and do not activate immune memory cells, so the immunization is considered passive.

What are the different types of vaccines?

A vaccine's composition influences the type and durability of the immune response it elicits. In this regard, vaccines are classified into one of six categories: live attenuated, inactivated (or killed), protein subunit, polysaccharide, polysaccharide conjugate, and recombinant.

Live attenuated virus vaccines are made from a virus that is weakened to the point that it cannot cause disease. As viruses, they act as parasites that depend on other cells to live. With live attenuated virus vaccines, a weakened virus enters a cell and reproduces just enough to induce an immune response but not enough to infect many other cells and cause illness. Three different methods are available to weaken viruses for vaccines. First, a virus could be grown in nonhuman cells. Viruses that infect humans grow best in human cells, so using nonhuman cells, such as chicken cells, as a growth medium ensures that the virus then will not reproduce very well in humans. This method is commonly used for chickenpox, measles, and mumps vaccines. A second method grows virus at temperatures lower than body temperature, thereby robbing the virus of its ability to reproduce well at body temperature. The third method combines elements of nonhuman and human viruses, retaining human virus components that induce the immune response while the nonhuman parts of the virus ensure the virus does not reproduce well enough to cause true infection and illness. This method is used for one of the rotavirus vaccines.

Inactivated or *killed vaccines* are made from a whole virus or bacteria that has been killed or neutralized through the application of a second substance—usually, a tiny amount of formaldehyde. Inactivated or killed viruses are not able to reproduce and cannot cause infection or disease, but because the body is still exposed to the whole virus, it is able to mount an immune response. The hepatitis A, polio, and most influenza vaccines utilize this method.

Protein subunit vaccines work by isolating the antigens or proteins on bacteria that are known to be important for inducing a protective immune response. Some protein subunit vaccines target antigens known to act as toxins. Diphtheria and tetanus vaccines, for example, are made by inactivating the toxins that these bacteria produce, creating inactivated toxins called *toxoids*. Pertussis vaccines are made from two to up to five different proteins that are either toxins or are part of the bacteria itself (compared to the 3,000 proteins contained in a whole pertussis bacterium). The inactivated proteins cannot cause infection or disease, but they will lead to an immune response to recognize and inactivate the bacteria or toxin when actual infection occurs.

Similar to protein subunit vaccines for bacteria, *recombinant vaccines* are made from individual viral proteins that are known to induce a protective immune response. To make recombinant vaccines, the gene that is responsible for making the selected protein is inserted into the DNA of a yeast cell. As the yeast reproduces, so too does the DNA, and the resulting protein is purified to make a vaccine. Both hepatitis B and HPV vaccines are made using this technique.

Polysaccharide vaccines target a certain group of bacteria that have a special capsule on their surface made of sugars or polysaccharides. Because their capsule is what the body interacts with first, it is also what the immune response targets. Thus, vaccines for encapsulated bacteria are made using this capsule rather than any proteins from the bacteria.

However, polysaccharide capsules do not induce immune memory well, nor do they work well in children younger than age 2 years. This is a problem because the bacteria with capsules—pneumococcus, meningococcus, and *Haemophilus influenzae* b (Hib)—can cause severe disease in young children. This led to the development of *conjugate vaccines*, in which the polysaccharide capsule is attached to a protein that is able to turn on memory cells.

Why are there so many types of vaccines?

Vaccine development has evolved as scientists learn more about how the body responds to certain pathogens and antigens; the ultimate goal is to produce antibodies that are specific to the pathogen but will not attack healthy cells in the body. These antibodies also need to target the right parts of the pathogen, both so the pathogen does not persist to cause infection and so the antibodies persist and are remembered as long as possible.

Why do most vaccines require more than one dose?

Some vaccines, particularly live attenuated virus vaccines, are efficient in generating a protective immune response because they turn on the immune system in a way that mimics natural infection. In these cases, one dose of a live virus vaccine is generally protective for most people. Inactivated or protein vaccines are not quite as efficient, so these vaccines require more than one dose to achieve complete protection. The additional vaccine doses, often called "boosters," help boost the immune response. The first dose is called a priming dose: Because it is the first time a person experiences the antigen, it is the first time the body starts to make the memory cells. The subsequent doses increase the number of memory cells and also help the body maintain circulating antibodies.

Besides antigens, what else are vaccines made of?

To keep vaccines safe and help increase their effectiveness, they may include other substances besides antigens. These include the following:

- Preservatives such as phenol and thimerosal (which is also known as ethylmercury) prevent vaccine contamination from any bacteria in the environment during and after production. These substances are especially important in preventing contamination after a vaccine vial has been opened for use. For this reason, preservatives are required in vials that contain more than one dose.
- Stabilizers, such as sugars, amino acids, or proteins, keep the vaccine functional for longer periods of time. Without stabilizers, vaccines' antigens would be degraded during

the temperature changes that take place during production, transportation, and storage.

- Inactivating agents such as formaldehyde inactivate viruses or bacterial toxins for inactivated virus or bacterial toxoid vaccines (see previous discussion about vaccine types). Formaldehyde is used during production of some vaccines to inactivate a virus or bacteria. Although the formaldehyde is removed after the virus or bacteria is inactivated, there can be a small residual amount left behind in production. The allowable residual is much lower than the amount of formaldehyde that naturally occurs within the body.

- Adjuvants, or substances that help enhance the immune response to vaccines, are especially important for elderly and immunocompromised patients who may have a weaker response to vaccination. Adjuvants also help enhance the immune response to vaccines that use only a few antigens; they are not needed in weakened or killed whole virus vaccines that induce a more complete immune response. Aluminum salts are most commonly used in US licensed vaccines. Aluminum is the most widely used vaccine additive because it helps boost the immune response, either by stimulating the uptake of antigens by immune cells or by slowing the release of an antigen at the site of injection to promote a more sustained antibody production. Vaccines containing aluminum adjuvants have been in use the longest and have a uniform track record of safety.

Adjuvants, preservatives, and inactivating agents are necessary to ensure safety and effectiveness in vaccine production. The fact that these substances include aluminum, formaldehyde, and thimerosal—substances that can be associated with toxicity above certain levels in the body—has raised safety concerns among some, particularly those who are hesitant about vaccines.

Even if these substances are necessary, are they safe?

There is no evidence that exposure to any of these substances in vaccines results in toxicity or illness. The use of any vaccine additive is regulated by the US Food and Drug Administration (FDA) and must follow strict requirements for allowable amounts. The details related to these additives are also a central focus of the licensing application for any vaccine, and these details cannot be changed without submitting an amendment to the FDA. As per federal requirements, the type and amount of all vaccine additives must be listed on a vaccine's label.

Heavy metals such as aluminum and mercury are present in the environment and can also be found in many foods that people eat. (Mercury, for example, can also be found in infant formula.) Human bodies excrete the heavy metals to which they are exposed, and every human has a small but detectable level of aluminum and mercury in his or her bloodstream at all times. The very small amounts of these substances found in vaccines do not increase these circulating levels, and the exposure that occurs with vaccination is negligible compared to what individuals encounter on a daily basis.

Formaldehyde, which is used to inactivate viruses or bacteria during vaccine manufacturing, has been shown to damage DNA in animal cells, which is the same process by which cancer cells are made. However, the tie between formaldehyde and damage to cell DNA is based only on animal models and laboratory experiments, and formaldehyde is not considered a human carcinogen. It is important to note that formaldehyde is a necessary component of human metabolic pathways, including DNA synthesis. For this reason, every individual has a detectable amount of formaldehyde in his or her bloodstream that far exceeds the amount found in vaccines.

What about thimerosal and autism?

Because mercury toxicity can affect the nervous system, there has been a concern that thimerosal (ethylmercury) could be linked to neurodevelopmental disorders such as autism (vaccines and autism are also discussed later). This concern arose after the 1998 publication of an article in the medical journal *The Lancet* in which British gastroenterologist Andrew Wakefield and colleagues presented a series of 12 patients who developed autistic behaviors and gastrointestinal symptoms after receiving the measles, mumps, and rubella (MMR) vaccine, which at the time contained thimerosal. The article hypothesized that the MMR vaccine may have prompted the production of antibodies that attacked the nervous system and led to the behavioral changes. On the coattails of the Wakefield study, others soon hypothesized that thimerosal could cause autism.

In the years that followed the publication of the Wakefield study, journalists and other scientists unearthed flaws in Wakefield et al.'s research, along with multiple professional conflicts of interest and ethics violations, that together discredited the study's findings and the authors' allegation of a link between MMR and neurodevelopmental disease (e.g., autism). In 2010, *The Lancet* took the extraordinary step of retracting the paper, with the journal's editor-in-chief telling *The Guardian* that the editorial board had been "deceived" by the authors' representation of their methods. Since initial publication of Wakefield et al.'s article and the journal's retraction, several subsequent studies have found no link between MMR, thimerosal, or any vaccine and autism.

Why was thimerosal removed from vaccines in 2001?

Wakefield et al.'s article prompted a public outcry about thimerosal's possible ties to autism, including demands for the removal of thimerosal from vaccines due to the concern for potential toxicity. Although there was no evidence of any adverse effects or mercury toxicity related to vaccination, the decision was made to remove thimerosal from all vaccines so that vaccination would not contribute to any exposure and, one could reasonably assume, to assuage any concerns and prevent vaccine acceptance from suffering. Today, thimerosal is used only in the multidose influenza vaccine in the United States. Because of the excellent preservative properties and lack of evidence of adverse effects, the World Health Organization continues to recommend thimerosal for use in multi-use vials in developing countries.

The bottom line is that using preservatives, stabilizers, and adjuvants allows us to use vaccines safely and effectively. Even if adjuvants such as aluminum were removed from vaccines, it would not decrease individuals' exposure to these substances in any significant way; it would, however, decrease vaccine effectiveness and safety.

Do some vaccines contain animal products?

Yes. Some vaccines contain weakened viruses, which can grow only in animal cells. The animal cells are used as a medium to grow the vaccine virus, which is then purified before being packaged as a vaccine. Purification takes place outside of the animal cell, but there may be very small amounts of animal protein or DNA in vaccines.

Gelatin, an animal product that is made from the skin or hooves of pigs, is also present in some vaccines. Gelatin is used as a stabilizing agent in some live virus vaccines (varicella, zoster, live attenuated influenza, and rabies), which may contain a sizable amount of it. This is an important consideration for those with severe allergy to gelatin—a very rare allergy (one case per 1 million doses) but still the most commonly identified cause of a severe allergy to vaccines. The presence of gelatin may also raise concerns for certain religious groups that have dietary restrictions regarding the ingestion of pig products. On this matter, religious leaders from most denominations have sanctioned the receipt of gelatin-containing vaccines because vaccination does not involve ingestion, and the modified gelatin used in vaccines is substantially different than natural gelatin.

Do vaccines use cells from aborted fetuses?

Some do, especially in cases in which the animal cells that are used to grow other vaccine viruses are insufficient. Because fetal cells act the same as human cells, they are more likely to support the replication of human viruses. They are also effectively sterile, having not been exposed to other viruses or bacteria as some animal cells can be. Because fetal cells reproduce indefinitely and without limit, they can be grown continually from a single source, and they are used extensively throughout biomedical research. In addition to vaccine development, human fetal cells have been used to develop treatments for HIV/AIDS, spinal cord injuries, cancer, and neurologic conditions such as Parkinson's disease and autism.

Fetal cells used for vaccine production today are grown from two different elective abortions that took place in Sweden and England in the 1960s. The fetal cells from Sweden were sent to the Wistar Institute in Philadelphia, where they were first used for rubella and rabies vaccines; this became known as the Wistar Institute-38 cell line. The cells from England were sent to the Medical Research Council and are known as MRC-5 cells. Currently, four vaccines are made using these cell lines: varicella, rubella, hepatitis A, and one of the rabies vaccines.

The use of fetal cells may pose a very difficult ethical dilemma for those who oppose abortion. In 2005, the Pontifical Academy for Life, a Vatican organization that considers bioethical intersections between science and faith, made a formal ruling on this issue, determining that the receipt of vaccines manufactured using fetal cells is acceptable: "Clearly the use of a vaccine in the present does not cause the one who is immunized to share in the immoral intention or action of those who carried out the abortion in the past."

2

A BRIEF HISTORY
OF VACCINES

The conceptual foundations of vaccination were first documented in ancient Greece, where physicians observed that getting infected with a virus could prevent reinfection with that same virus. In 900–1000 A.D., early forms of the modern vaccine were developed in China when physicians first noted that people exposed to smallpox scab tissue would be protected from getting smallpox or would develop milder disease. Smallpox scabs were often crushed into powder and inhaled through the nose, and similar interventions were employed for hundreds of years thereafter in Asia, the Middle East, and Africa. In 1715, Lady Mary Montagu, the wife of England's ambassador to Turkey, learned about the practice after she developed smallpox and was in search of a way to protect her children. She is credited with bringing inoculation to England when she had a physician inoculate her 2-year-old child in 1721.

However, it was not until the early 18th century that the first vaccine came to the United States.

When was the first vaccination delivered in the United States?

The Boston smallpox epidemic of 1721 began when smallpox was brought to US shores on a ship from the Caribbean. Although it was not the first smallpox epidemic in colonial America, it was the first time an intervention was attempted to prevent disease. The intervention occurred through a practice called *inoculation*, also known as *variolation*. At the time, the use of inoculation was somewhat speculative because it occurred long before there was a good understanding of the multiple pathways of the immune system or even germ theory.

What is inoculation?

The Merriam–Webster Dictionary defines inoculation as "the introduction of a pathogen or antigen into a living organism to stimulate the production of antibodies." During the 1721 smallpox epidemic, fluid from an infected individual's smallpox pustule was introduced to healthy individuals through a small cut in the skin. The person who received the inoculation would develop smallpox but generally a milder case. The individual would then be protected from subsequent infections through antibody protection, although the role of antibodies was not understood at the time.

The introduction of inoculation was fraught with controversy. Cotton Mather, a Boston minister known for his championing role in the Salem witch trials, made the first call for inoculation in response to the 1721 epidemic.

Mather first learned of inoculation and its benefits from both incoming slaves who had the procedure performed in their home country and texts from the Royal Society of Medicine in Britain. Mather had previously portrayed smallpox in religious terms—an act of Providence or a reflection of man's sin—but during the 1721 epidemic, he chose instead to intervene, citing the will of God.

Interestingly, Mather found almost no support within the medical community, save for one physician named Zabdiel Boylston, who agreed to offer inoculation. By the end of the epidemic, Boylston had inoculated 248 patients, mostly in secret. However, by the time the next smallpox epidemic hit Boston in 1730, the practice was beginning to gain traction.

Why the controversy?

From a medical perspective, although it had been practiced in many countries throughout the world and was described in medical texts, the available literature did not provide much evidence of the efficacy of inoculation or its safety when it was first introduced. People who developed smallpox after inoculation could still infect others, so quarantine was important. It was difficult for many people to accept making themselves intentionally ill as a preventive measure: People accepted some interventions, many dangerous, to treat an illness, but it was more difficult to accept a new intervention that made them willfully ill (albeit less ill than if they contracted smallpox through traditional contagion routes) when they were otherwise feeling well. There were also those who feared that inoculation could lead to chronic health problems and others who had moral and spiritual reservations. Many of these sentiments resonate today among individuals who have concerns about vaccines.

Controversies aside, infections associated with inoculation appeared to be less severe and provided protection from subsequent infection. Adoption remained slow, but the medical community did eventually embrace it, sometimes adding a string of preparatory (and largely unnecessary) interventions prior to inoculation. In 1757, an English surgeon and his son developed a simpler procedure (use of a thin needle rather than a lancet) and established a society of 200 inoculation practitioners worldwide. Despite this organization, inoculation remained against the law in many colonies through the Revolutionary War, but it was practiced extensively in larger cities such as Philadelphia and Boston.

How did we get from inoculation to vaccination?

Again, smallpox. In 1796, Edward Jenner, a doctor in the English countryside, was treating a milkmaid who claimed that she never got smallpox because she had been exposed to cowpox, a viral disease similar to smallpox but milder and less common. Cowpox was mostly limited to farmworkers who acquired the disease through cow udders. It was not as severe as smallpox, but it still caused inflamed joints, skin ulcers, fever, and limb pain. As opposed to smallpox, cowpox did not cause disfigurement or death.

Jenner's first field experiment was to find a group of farmers who had a history of cowpox and inoculate them with smallpox; he did so, and none of the farmers developed smallpox. In May 1796, he performed the ultimate test: He took fluid from lesions of a milkmaid who had just developed cowpox and then inoculated a young boy with it. Several weeks later, Jenner inoculated the boy with smallpox and nothing happened; the boy never showed symptoms of the more serious disease. Jenner had demonstrated that cowpox gave immunity against smallpox. By 1801, 100,000 people throughout Europe had received the first cowpox-based smallpox vaccine.

When did smallpox vaccine come to the United States?

Interestingly, cowpox did not affect cows in the United States, so there was no access to the fluid needed to make the vaccine that had been successful in the United Kingdom. Some domestic doctors received samples from the United Kingdom, but this limited supply could not keep pace with the massive demand. This paved the way for fraudulent and black-market vaccines, the use of which led people who thought they were protected to still contract smallpox. The proliferation of these incidents almost completely halted smallpox vaccination in the United States until Thomas Jefferson intervened to establish the widespread import of cowpox fluid (or *vaccinia*). He also worked with doctors to conduct studies to show that vaccination was indeed effective (see https://www.historyofvaccines.org/timeline).

How well did this early vaccine really work?

Today, we can hypothesize that the cowpox virus was similar to smallpox and could therefore lead to cross-reactivity—that is, the antibodies made to fight cowpox also recognized and worked against smallpox.

Neither Jenner nor his contemporaries had any firm concept of bacteria or viruses, and presumably they understood little about the mechanisms behind their observations. Their evidence was based on the number of vaccinated individuals who developed (or did not develop) smallpox after exposure. Although the vaccine did prevent disease, the lack of understanding led to errors in vaccine administration, including use of nonliving virus (which would produce no immune reaction and would provide no protection) and patients' development of skin infections from bacteria or tetanus due to vaccine contamination. The occurrence of these problems lessened as the medical and scientific community learned more.

What was the public response to the new vaccine?

Support for vaccination developed more slowly in the United States than in the United Kingdom. By the early 19th century, US vaccine uptake was mostly limited to larger cities, in which the population was at higher risk for smallpox epidemics compared to rural communities. In response to frequent outbreaks, Boston was the first US city to enact a mandatory vaccination law in 1827, and Massachusetts was the first state to do so in 1855.

As the century progressed, the US Civil War and the Franco-Prussian War offered evidence on both continents for the importance of vaccines: Armies that required vaccination had lower numbers of smallpox cases and deaths compared to civilian populations or armies that did not require vaccination. This led to a more concerted post-war effort to ensure a stable vaccine supply and to mandate vaccination. However, enforcement remained uneven, and because vaccine supply was inconsistent, acceptance of such laws was uneven as well.

In Europe, where cowpox was common, vaccine farms were created to help ensure a more stable and consistently effective supply of vaccines that did not require fluid from lesions of infected people. This practice soon caught on in the United States as well, and throughout most of the 19th century, smallpox vaccines were created "direct from the cow" on vaccine farms via fluid recovered directly from cowpox lesions on calves. Initially, the United States imported these cowpox strains—the first to be widely propagated was called the Beaugency vaccine strain from France. Eventually, vaccine farms were established in the United States after 1870, when a physician from Boston imported the Beaugency vaccine strain and inoculated several cows. Over time, the practice was upgraded to include techniques that minimized risk of contamination from other bacteria. Despite these improvements, most people generally avoided vaccination until there was an epidemic.

The introduction of Jenner's vaccine was also countered by the emergence of the first anti-vaccine movement. The 1871 Vaccination Act in Britain, which required poor individuals to be vaccinated or risk fines or property loss, gave rise to the National Anti-Vaccination League, which opposed compulsory vaccination based on concerns that centered on vaccine safety and effectiveness.

In the United States, an organized anti-vaccine movement took longer to develop. Many individuals were wary of compulsory vaccination programs, and local anti-vaccination societies emerged without much widespread organization or membership. It was not until 1906 when John Pitcairn, a self-made millionaire and Swedenborgian (a 19th-century Christian denomination that believed vaccination represented contamination of the soul), founded the Anti-Vaccination League of Pennsylvania, the first anti-vaccination organization with significant financial resources and organization. Pitcairn's activism was spurred by anger over compulsory laws that required vaccination for everyone, even those who opposed it due to their religious beliefs. (Note that at the time of Pitcairn's efforts, a less severe strain of smallpox had become more prevalent in many communities. Therefore, there was less fear of smallpox, which made compulsory vaccination seem less necessary and more objectionable to some individuals.)

Pitcairn's efforts to block compulsory laws in Pennsylvania were not successful, and he went on to help establish the Anti-Vaccination League of America in 1908, an organization whose main goal was to "promote universal acceptance of the principle that health is nature's greatest safeguard against disease and that therefore no State has the right to demand of anyone the impairment of his or her health." The Anti-Vaccination League of America attracted some vocal activists and focused its efforts on blocking compulsory vaccination laws. Many of the beliefs that fueled the group's arguments still resonate today. Some in the organization rejected the idea that diseases were caused by specific germs that needed to be prevented, arguing instead that diseases were a symptom of uncleanliness or poor health. Others considered vaccination to be ineffective and unsanitary, and they emphasized the importance of having control over one's own body. Vaccination was also considered an example of public health and medicine overstepping its bounds: "Be your own doctor" is a statement from one 1911 League advertisement. Pitcairn and the group's leadership lobbied state legislatures and engaged in public debates about vaccination. These efforts led to the defeat of mandatory vaccination legislation in some states in the 1910s, but the group began to lose momentum by the 1920s as vaccination and other public health prevention measures successfully prevented diseases such as tuberculosis, diphtheria, and tetanus. Vaccine technology had also begun to improve, which in turn increased confidence in vaccine safety.

How did the public health community make early vaccines safer?

Smallpox vaccines were born of an imperfect science that reflected the limited knowledge of their era. The flaws of this first class of vaccines came to a head during the 1901–1904 smallpox epidemic that affected cities and states throughout the United States. After widespread compulsory immunization campaigns were initiated to stop disease transmission, an outbreak of tetanus deaths among vaccinated patients in Philadelphia, Camden, Cleveland, and Atlantic City quickly followed—all related to vaccines produced by one manufacturer. This highlighted the lack of oversight on vaccine production and stirred a public distrust for the safety of vaccine science. An ensuing investigation led by physician Joseph McFarland found that contamination may have been due to inadequate use of glycerin, which was added to vaccines during that time to kill potentially contaminating bacteria. In July 1902, Congress passed the US Biologics Control Act, which regulated vaccines that moved across state lines; ensuing regulations required testing for tetanus and other bacteria. These laws were not easy to enforce, but more stringent requirements led to fewer (and better) licensed vaccine manufacturers. In 1906, Congress followed with the Pure Food and Drug Act of 1906, which laid the groundwork for the US Food and Drug Administration.

As the regulatory infrastructure for vaccines came on line in the United States, the modern vaccine movement began amid a flurry of scientific advancements. Louis Pasteur's germ theory, which is founded on principles that infectious diseases are caused by microorganisms such as bacteria and viruses, became widely accepted. Pasteur also showed that germs did not appear spontaneously, as was the widespread belief at the time, but rather that they are in the environment and air. Pasteur also found that if he boiled liquid to kill any germs (a process that became known as pasteurization) and sealed the container, no germs would then grow. This idea of killing contaminating germs, or making something "aseptic," led to the development of techniques to make surgery and food safer.

What were some of the key developments in vaccine science during this time?

One of the most important developments in vaccine science was that of *attenuation*, in which a virus or bacteria is weakened so that it cannot cause disease but can still lead to an immune response and subsequent protection. Pasteur demonstrated attenuation through the development of a cholera vaccine for chickens in which he grew the cholera microbe in an acidic culture media (setting); the acidic environment appeared to weaken the virus without rendering it unusable in a vaccine. A Pasteur contemporary, Henri Toussaint, developed an anthrax vaccine using similar methods. These vaccines proved effective in laboratory and animal experiments, but they were not immediately tested on humans.

This changed in 1885 when Pasteur also used the attenuation approach to develop a rabies vaccine and administered it to two 14-year-old boys who had been bitten by rabid dogs—his first use of an attenuated vaccine in humans. Both boys survived, but the experiment was at first largely condemned by both the public and the medical community. However, the boys' survival eventually gave rise to more volunteers for the vaccine among people who had been bitten, and their uniform survival garnered support and praise for Pasteur.

The sum of all of these discoveries was an overall boom in the development of new vaccines and the identification of ways to make vaccines safer.

How did vaccine development begin to take off?

The end of the 19th century brought huge leaps in vaccine discovery and the accompanying practices that made vaccines more effective and safer for use. As Pasteur developed his attenuated rabies vaccine, other groups of scientists found ways to make vaccines using killed viruses or bacteria. These discoveries led to the first human vaccines for typhoid, plague, and cholera between 1879 and 1897.

At the turn of the 20th century, scientists discovered antitoxins in the serum (a blood component) of animals that had been infected with certain bacteria—that is, diphtheria and tetanus. The antitoxins were found to neutralize the diphtheria and tetanus bacteria when they were grown in a laboratory. This led to the discovery of how antibodies interact with specific antigens. It also led to the commercial production of antitoxin containing animal serum (from horses and rabbits) to help protect exposed people from developing disease. Scientists began calling rabbit serum "immune serum," and the term *immunization* was born.

What were some other important developments for making vaccines?

The first vaccines were made from either attenuated or killed bacteria or viruses: viruses had to be grown in animals (Table 2.1). In the 1920s, a husband–wife team of scientists introduced tissue culture, and then in 1931, E. W. Goodpasture introduced the use of eggs, or chick embryos, to grow viruses. The use of chick embryos proved to be a faster and safer methodology and facilitated the development of many new vaccines, including influenza vaccines. In 1949, a new technique called cell culture was introduced. This meant that viruses could be grown even more easily in a laboratory, revolutionizing vaccine development.

The next major development was facilitated by a growing understanding of the relationship between specific antigen and antibody. With this knowledge, scientists began developing vaccines made from specific proteins or the outer carbohydrate capsule of bacteria, leading to many of the vaccine types described in Chapter 1. In the 1980s, a group of investigators from California took this a step further and developed

Table 2.1 Timeline of Vaccine Development

Time Period	Vaccine Type	Diseases Targeted
1920s–1930s	Live-attenuated	Tuberculosis, yellow fever
	Killed whole virus/ bacteria	Pertussis, influenza, typhus
	Protein	Diphtheria and tetanus toxoid
1950s–1960s	Live attenuated	Oral polio, measles, mumps
	Killed whole virus/ bacteria	Injected polio
1970s–1980s	Live attenuated	Typhoid
	Killed whole virus/ bacteria	Rabies (cell culture), tick-borne encephalitis
	Protein	*Pneumococcus* polysaccharide *Meningococcus* polysaccharide *Haemophilus influenzae* b polysaccharide and conjugate
	Recombinant	Hepatitis B surface antigen
1990s	Attenuated	Varicella, rotavirus
	Killed whole virus/ bacteria	Hepatitis A, cholera
	Protein	Typhoid Acellular pertussis Meningococcal conjugate (group C)
	Recombinant	Cholera
2000s	Attenuated	Cold-adapted influenza, rotavirus, zoster
	Killed whole virus/ bacteria	Japanese encephalitis, cholera
	Protein	Pneumococcal conjugate, meningococcal conjugate (ACWY)
	Recombinant	Human papillomavirus

recombinant vaccines in which genes that are responsible for making proteins are placed inside yeast cells. With this new genetic material, the yeast make these proteins, which can then be used in a vaccine.

What was the impact of vaccine introduction on disease incidence?

The impact of vaccines increased once there was an immunization program to structuralize vaccine delivery, particularly for children, for whom most early vaccines were intended. Once children were able to receive vaccines on a large scale, the incidence, or number of new cases, of vaccine-preventable diseases began to decrease very significantly (Table 2.2).

However, vaccine impact does depend on how well the vaccine covers the pathogen. For example, some viruses and bacteria, such as pneumococcus and meningococcus, have several different types or groups that may circulate in a community. A vaccine may target only some of the types, so there can still be cases caused by types not covered by the vaccine. Immunization rates and the communicability of the pathogen are also important for vaccine impact because of herd immunity (see Chapter 1).

What about vaccine introduction in other countries?

The practice of inoculation was first documented in countries in Asia and Africa, followed by Europe. As inoculation became more common in European countries, the practice was more widely exported to these nations' colonies (in some cases, to make countries safe for colonizers or as part of a "civilizing

Table 2.2 Vaccine-preventable Disease Annual Incidence Before and After Vaccine Introduction

Vaccine-Preventable Disease	Pre-vaccine Era Number of Cases/Year	Reported Cases as of January 1, 2016
Measles	530,217	667
Diphtheria	21,053	1
Varicella	4,085,120	151,149
Pertussis	200,752	32,971
Polio	16,316	0
Rubella	47,745	6
Mumps	162,344	1,223

mission"). Vaccination also spread to other countries from China, including Korea and Japan. Korea established its first cowpox vaccination clinics in the 1880s and introduced cholera and typhoid vaccines at the turn of the century. India was one of the first countries to practice inoculation and first introduced Jenner's smallpox vaccine in 1802; until 1850, however, India had to import it from England. By the early 20th century, India began its own production of vaccines against smallpox, cholera, typhoid, and plague, but it faced challenges in distributing vaccines to the population.

In Africa, ethnic groups across several regions used smallpox inoculation before the practice was introduced to Europe and the United States. As mentioned previously, Cotton Mather first learned of inoculation from an African slave. However, the use of modern vaccines in Africa was largely part of European colonialism: By 1938, there were eight European medical research laboratories (including the Pasteur Institute) in North and sub-Saharan Africa to support vaccine development for distribution in the region. In general, countries adopted newly developed vaccines as resources allowed for importation or production, storage, and distribution. This meant that global vaccine uptake was uneven, at least until coordinated efforts to achieve smallpox eradication were established and the subsequent development of the Expanded Programme on Immunization by the World Health Organization in 1974. This initiative was created to help ensure that all children have access to vaccines protecting against six of the most common and deadly childhood diseases—tuberculosis, tetanus, measles, diphtheria, pertussis, and polio—and it helps support immunization programs in low- and middle-income countries (see Chapter 4).

3

VACCINE DEVELOPMENT

Vaccine development is a long process that requires numerous highly regulated steps, many years, and significant scientific and financial resources. Given the breadth of infections that affect children and adults, how are decisions made about which ones to prevent with vaccination? Once vaccine development begins, what exactly happens and who is responsible?

To begin this discussion, it is important to consider how the factors that drive vaccine development have changed in recent decades. In the early to mid-20th century, when vaccine-preventable diseases were still highly prevalent, the development of new vaccines was dictated by how quickly the new vaccines could reduce disease burden to make a significant impact on children's health. Since then, amid widespread availability of vaccines, the occurrence of vaccine-preventable diseases has decreased, and urgency is no longer the primary driver. Vaccine development now places greater emphasis on *benefit over risk*. Today's regulatory environment places as much emphasis on how safe a vaccine is for healthy people as on a vaccine's capacity to prevent disease, and accordingly the requirements for vaccine production have shifted. Today, there is a very high bar for the demonstration of vaccine safety, enforced through regulations and quality control measures that guide vaccine development and manufacturing.

As with all facets of health care, vaccine development has also faced a growing emphasis on cost-effectiveness. Because immunization programs have expanded throughout the world, they require more resources to ensure supply and distribution and in turn are subject to an added layer of scrutiny related to production scale and financing. This has particular implications for newer vaccine technologies, which have allowed for the development of more effective vaccines and targeting of new diseases, albeit at a higher price. Immunization programs must accordingly consider the potential costs and benefits of using new vaccines—for example, How many people need to be vaccinated to prevent one case? and How much will it cost an immunization program to prevent each case? This market calculus also influences how vaccine manufacturers develop and price new vaccines, as they consider the potential demand and reception for a vaccine before allocating the investment for its development.

What factors influence which vaccines get developed?

The decision to proceed with the scientific phase of vaccine development begins with perceived need or public health importance. These needs are generally measured by epidemiologists—scientists who study how infections spread, who becomes infected, and who is most at risk. Because vaccines are administered to groups of individuals, vaccine scientists may prioritize infections that affect a large proportion of the population, or they may prioritize infections that result in severe disease. They may also consider the availability of other methods to prevent infection. The evaluation of disease burden may include consideration of the number of cases, the impact of illness on quality of life, the death rates due to the disease, and the cost to the health care system.

A disease does not have to occur frequently to be considered "high burden." Uncommon diseases that have a high fatality rate are just as likely to be considered high burden as diseases that are relatively uncommon but highly contagious, meaning that when they do occur, they can rapidly result in an outbreak. As a contemporary example, consider the Ebola outbreak in West Africa in 2014 and 2015. Ebola virus is not a common infection, and it is generally localized in isolated regions. However, because it spreads easily and causes a severe infection that produces a high mortality rate, it carries a potential to affect large swaths of people relatively quickly. After the initial outbreak of Ebola in West Africa, prevention interventions such as the use of protective equipment helped prevent some new infections (transmission of Ebola requires exposure to body fluid from an infected individual), but preventing all contact through such methods proved impossible. Combined with the absence of any readily available and effective treatment for Ebola, vaccine development became an important priority to stop the outbreak.

This example also highlights the importance of knowing as much as possible about the pathogen, including how it causes infection and who is most likely to be infected. To develop an effective vaccine, scientists need to have some idea of which part of a bacteria or virus stimulates the human immune system and leads to immune memory. Without this understanding, it is difficult to know where to begin for vaccine development.

Cost considerations have begun to figure more prominently into vaccine development. Public health systems now consider investment costs versus public health benefit to prioritize vaccine development. There are tools to help provide structure to such assessments, including the World Health Organization's CHOICE (CHOosing Interventions that are Cost-Effective) project. A common way that cost-effectiveness is measured is by quality-adjusted life years (QALYs). This is a measure that tries to quantify the effects of a vaccine on health-related quality of life. It is a standardized measure, meaning that it is calculated using a set formula. Policymakers can then compare QALYs gained by vaccines across different diseases.

Before investing in the development of a specific or targeted vaccine, vaccine companies consider the likely return on their upfront investment and whether market reception will allow for the vaccine's continued production and development. For vaccine manufacturers, the market for a new vaccine is largely measured by whether the vaccine will receive uptake from national immunization programs. The companies also assess the ability of these immunization programs to purchase the vaccines, which can be difficult because vaccine distribution largely occurs through departments in the public sector that have limited budgets. Such considerations are particularly important for vaccines that would be used predominately in resource-limited settings, such as a malaria or cholera vaccine. Humanitarian nonprofit organizations that help low-resource countries purchase vaccines therefore have a substantial role in vaccine development: By providing vaccine manufacturers with reliable, projectable markets (and revenue), these foundations can influence vaccine development and pricing in a way that makes vaccines accessible to both resource-limited and wealthy countries.

Once a decision to proceed with vaccine development is made, what are the steps needed to bring a vaccine from an idea to production?

The first stage of vaccine development is grounded in research—understanding how a particular pathogen interacts with the immune system. This is carried out through basic science research in laboratories, often by researchers from universities but also at pharmaceutical companies or nonprofit organizations. The goal is to determine which part of a bacteria or virus sparks the immune system to make protective antibodies. This is done by performing experiments using test tubes or in animal studies. Many vaccine candidates do not progress beyond this stage because they do not appear to spark the immune system well enough or it appears that they would not be tolerated very well. If the vaccine candidate does seem promising, it moves on to the first real phase of vaccine development—preclinical development.

During preclinical development, the antigens to be used in the vaccine are isolated and purified. Much attention is paid to the properties of the antigen and the scientists' ability to reliably and repeatedly produce it, and this initial groundwork also involves multiple quality-assurance tests. Scientists also need to be able to demonstrate a mechanism of action (how the vaccine works with the immune system) and evaluate both the immune response and potential side effects. This is generally done through animal testing. By examining the immune response and safety in animals, researchers can determine how the vaccine may work in people, which in turn can help them identify a safe starting dose. Preclinical studies may not take place with a vaccine manufacturer; these investigations are more often carried out by researchers at universities, government research labs, or biotech companies.

Once these initial steps have been acceptably passed, a vaccine candidate can move to studies in people, known as *clinical trials*. However, most candidate vaccines do not move past preclinical development.

What is required for clinical studies?

According to the US Food, Drug, and Cosmetic Act (1938), it is illegal to give any experimental substance, including a candidate vaccine, to humans until it has been reviewed and approved by the US Food and Drug Administration (FDA) to ensure it has promise to be effective and is relatively safe. This cannot take place until an Investigational New Drug (IND) application is submitted to and approved by the FDA. These applications define the identity and purity of the antigen, in addition to the amount of it that is to be included in the proposed vaccine. The applications also include results from preclinical studies about safety and the mechanism of action for the vaccine. Last, the IND also needs to show that vaccine development will follow good manufacturing practices that require multiple quality control and quality assurance steps. Once this is complete and the application is accepted, vaccine development can move into clinical development.

INDs are generally submitted by vaccine manufacturers that have the infrastructure and resources needed to fulfill required manufacturing practices and produce test vaccines for clinical studies. Vaccine manufacturers, called *sponsors* at this stage, will then contract with research institutions to carry out the clinical studies. The sponsor provides the vaccine, whereas the researcher is responsible for recruiting patients, collecting data, and reporting back to the sponsor, which in turn then presents the data to the FDA. This is a highly regulated process governed by a series of federal laws aimed at protecting individuals participating in research studies and safety.

Clinical development is divided into three phases. Phase I evaluates safety and immune response in small groups of adult volunteers. In this phase, multiple studies may evaluate different vaccine formulations to determine which gives the best immune response with the least side effects. For a vaccine being designed for children, Phase I studies will still start with adults and then gradually include increasingly younger people.

In Phase II, a candidate vaccine's safety and immunogenicity (ability to provoke an immune response) are evaluated in a larger group of several hundred volunteers. These trials may also begin to measure efficacy—the difference in disease incidence or infection between vaccinated and unvaccinated individuals. These outcomes will be considered for each specific antigen dose and immunization schedule.

Based on the results from these studies, vaccine developers will prepare for larger Phase III trials, which focus solely on efficacy. As such, these trials usually involve an even larger number of participants, especially for infections that may not be very common, and place continued emphasis on safety and consistency across lots (batches) of vaccines.

In both Phase II and Phase III, participants who receive the vaccine are compared to participants who receive a placebo. Phase II and III trials may also evaluate how well the vaccine works and whether there are changes to the safety profile when the candidate vaccine is administered with other vaccines. This is especially important if the new vaccine is proposed to be added to an existing immunization schedule and would therefore be administered at the same time as other vaccines.

Is there a similar process in other countries?

In the European Union (EU), there are three different licensing procedures. The first is centralized, in which all preclinical, technical, and clinical information is reviewed by the European Medicines Agency (EMA) followed by the Committee for Medicinal Products for Human Use. If both bodies approve, the vaccine is usually licensed by the European Commission and can be given in any EU country. There is also a mutual recognition process through which a vaccine may have approval in one state and the manufacturer can request mutual recognition in other EU states.

However, even if a vaccine has been licensed in other countries and is being widely used in these countries, it cannot be given in the United States until it has been reviewed and approved by the FDA. This requirement made headlines in 2013 and 2014 when outbreaks of meningococcal B disease on two US college campuses prompted calls for the meningococcal B vaccine that had been approved and in use in several countries, including those in the EU, but had not been approved by the FDA. To use the meningococcal B vaccine to stop the outbreaks, a special application had to be filed to request emergency approval even though it was a vaccine used routinely in other countries.

In countries that do not have highly developed regulatory agencies, approval in the country of manufacture is generally considered sufficient. For organizations such as UNICEF and the United Nations that administer large numbers of vaccines across a wide range of countries, the World Health Organization oversees a prequalification procedure through which it reviews and determines the acceptability of any vaccine purchased and administered by the nonprofit agencies.

To address variability in standards across different countries, the International Conference on Harmonisation's *ICH Harmonised Tripartite Guideline: Guideline for Good Clinical Practice* (more succinctly, "the GCP") was published in the 1990s to establish an international standard for the design, conduct, monitoring, and reporting of clinical research of investigational drugs, including vaccines. Standardization of procedures for the clinical development of vaccines was meant to increase the integrity of results from clinical trials that could then be applied to licensure applications across different countries. Of note, the United States has not officially signed on to the GCP, instead publishing its own similar standards as part of the *Code of Federal Regulations*. However, the GCP is generally followed in the development of new vaccines because it may be a requirement of the vaccine manufacturer sponsoring clinical development and planning to distribute the vaccine globally.

Are there protections for people who participate in clinical trials?

The FDA has strict standards for protecting study participants that must be met before the results of a clinical trial are accepted. These standards are based on international standards that apply to any research studies involving people—a set of rules that were first developed after World War II and the Nuremberg Trials in response to the abuse of human subjects during wartime experiments on concentration camp prisoners. The *Nuremberg Code* (1947) became the foundation for ethical principles for research involving people, followed by the *Declaration of Helsinki* in 1964. In 1976, these principles were codified as formal regulations in the United States as the *Belmont Report*.

The *Belmont Report* identifies three key principles: justice, beneficence (or do no harm), and respect for persons. In practice, this means that participation in a study requires informed consent. Informed consent must include adequate information about study goals and procedures with confirmation of understanding and voluntariness. All study proposals must include an assessment of risks and benefits and demonstrate that any potential risks are outweighed by potential benefit. Without this assessment, a study cannot be justified. Last, selection of study subjects must be done fairly. To ensure that these principles are carried out, most institutions that conduct research maintain an institutional review board, which is a governing body that reviews and must approve all protocols involving research with humans.

How many people are involved in vaccine trials?

The average size of a Phase I trial is small and may include only 20–80 individuals; Phase II studies encompass several hundred people. Phase III trials are even larger, from thousands to tens of thousands, with a goal of simulating and measuring population-level impact on disease rates and safety. The size of Phase II trials varies based on how frequently the disease or safety event occurs: For outcomes that do not occur frequently, larger numbers of subjects are required. For example, during rotavirus vaccine development, manufacturers were particularly interested in determining whether the vaccine increased the risk of intussusception—a twisting of the intestines that results in blockage and occurs at a rate of 1 in 10,000 infants in the general population. Intussusception had been identified as an uncommon adverse event associated with an earlier rotavirus vaccine that was approved in 1998 and subsequently removed from the market. At that time, reports of intussusception among recently vaccinated healthy infants prompted closer investigation that found an increased risk that could lead to an additional one or two cases for every 10,000 doses given. Because this was an uncommon adverse event, it was not identified during the pre-licensure clinical trials which included approximately 7,000 infants. Thus, for the new rotavirus vaccines, larger trials were required to ensure intussusception would be picked up. This required trials with 60,000 infants to be able to simulate a risk similar to that for the general population.

What happens after clinical development is complete?

Once all three phases are complete, results are submitted for licensure to the relevant governing body. To succeed, the candidate vaccine must demonstrate a clear clinical benefit with minimal risks. Patient safety is monitored throughout each step of the process, and study participants (those who receive the vaccine as well as those who receive the placebo) are required to report any side effects that occur during their participation in the vaccine trials. Licensure review also includes a review of manufacturing and labeling processes to ensure consistency and adherence to quality controls.

Once a vaccine is licensed, it is available for uptake by immunization programs, which means that the vaccine can be recommended and administered to even larger groups of people. The vaccine's monitoring is not finished; at this point, a vaccine enters "Phase IV," or a period of post-licensure surveillance. This includes monitoring for adverse events as the vaccine is administered to populations, as well as effectiveness studies to monitor how well the vaccine works to reduce disease in vaccinated individuals and populations. Having a vaccine available for use among the public also allows for surveillance of how a vaccine works "outside the laboratory"—for example, when administered on a schedule other than the recommended schedule or in individuals with or without a history of medical problems who would not have been allowed to participate in the clinical trials made up of healthy participants.

What evidence do vaccine developers search for during development to show that a vaccine works?

This is one of the challenges in vaccine development. Initially, scientists look for evidence of an immune response, or antibody production. It is important to note that *immune response* and *antibody production* can be different in this context: Some infections or diseases have known antibody levels that equate to protection, whereas for others, antibody levels do not necessarily correspond to protection, and other parts of the immune response may be involved. In the latter case, it is optimal to be able to measure actual impact on clinical outcomes—for example, the frequency of a disease's incidence in a population of people vaccinated against it. Of course, this requires larger trials to be able to observe enough people who could develop the disease.

In postlicensing surveillance, vaccine surveillance is conducted by both vaccine manufacturers and public health agencies. Vaccine manufacturers follow the impact on disease rates over time in Phase IV studies, whereas public agencies follow the epidemiology of vaccine-preventable diseases after a vaccine is added to immunization programs.

How long does this whole process take—from the first exploratory study to licensure of a new vaccine?

Vaccine research and development leading up to (and not including) submission for approval usually takes 10–15 years. For some vaccines, the development process has required more than 20 years. Of this, the exploratory and preclinical studies in laboratories and animals can take 3–6 years, and clinical trials require an additional several years so that there is enough time to observe study participants for a sufficient duration to determine how well the vaccine works and to ensure it is safe. After the vaccine portfolio is submitted to the FDA or the EMA, review and subsequent licensure generally takes approximately 10–12 months.

Is a vaccine ever approved or used without following these steps?

In general, any medication (including a new vaccine) requires approval before it can enter a given market, and this is certainly the case in the United States. However, in some instances, these steps can be shortened, typically in cases in which there is an urgent need to stop an outbreak. Such was the case in 2009 during the novel H1N1 influenza pandemic: Waiting for a year would have resulted in a significant delay in being able to prevent the disease and stop its transmission, which in light of the public health risks was deemed unacceptable. Thus, for cases of acute outbreaks such as H1N1 or Ebola, licensing agencies have alternate pathways for a more rapid review.

The EU has two alternate pathways. The first is called a "mock-up" procedure, in which an influenza strain is identified as having the potential to cause a future pandemic and vaccine research is undertaken preemptively. If a pandemic does occur, a more specific or modified pandemic influenza strain can be substituted in the mock-up vaccine, and the development of the vaccine proceeds with the benefit of groundwork already being laid. Mock-up influenza vaccines were converted to production in the EU during the 2009 H1N1 pandemic. There are currently four mock-up vaccines against H5N1 (avian) influenza strains that have mock-up approval and could move to production if there is an H5N1 pandemic.

The second pathway in the EU is called the "emergency procedure," which allows for fast-track review and approval (approximately 2 months) of a new vaccine developed after a pandemic has started. In these instances, vaccine manufacturers must still submit a full application, but they can submit the individual elements on a rolling basis, as they are available. If the review shows that benefits outweigh risks, conditional approval may be given, with full approval contingent upon receipt of all data when they are available. In the interim, the pathway will allow the vaccine to be used during the pandemic. This pathway was also used during the 2009 H1N1 influenza pandemic for two pandemic influenza vaccines.

The United States also has procedures in place for rapid approval of pandemic (and season-specific) influenza vaccines. In these cases, vaccine manufacturers can use an existing licensing application (including specifications for things such as manufacturing) for new, seasonal influenza vaccines. This allows the applications to focus on efficacy and safety of pandemic and seasonal influenza vaccines, resulting in a faster review.

If these pathways were not in place, it would be difficult to ensure availability of new vaccines in response to outbreaks.

Who is involved in all of these steps from conceptualization to development?

Both conceptualization and development of a vaccine involve several factions of players. Universities and research institutes are largely responsible for carrying out basic and clinical research that informs vaccine development. Here, scientists with expertise in fields such as microbiology, immunology, and virology may perform the investigations to identify antigens that would be good candidates for vaccines. These academic researchers may be funded by federal agencies such as the National Institutes of Health (NIH) or the Centers for Disease Control and Prevention (CDC) to build foundational knowledge on disease pathophysiology, epidemiology, and immunology. The NIH also maintains its own foundational laboratories and investigators, which are funded by the US government. In addition, the US Department of Defense and the US Agency for International Development may also support the development of vaccines, particularly those for individuals participating in military operations internationally or for young children in developing countries.

Once this basic research is complete, researchers will collaborate with a pharmaceutical company for clinical studies and the other components of vaccine development. Although advances in immunology and microbiology have expanded vaccine manufacturers' ability to make vaccines, production is not easy (as detailed previously): The bar is very high for a vaccine to be licensed, and the production processes are tightly regulated. A pharmaceutical company needs to be able to do all of the following, and meet the rigorous standards of regulating agencies in doing so, in order to be successful:

- Produce the antigen or active component of a vaccine
- Stabilize the antigen
- Produce the antigen cleanly (i.e., without by-products that cause environmental or bodily harm)
- Package the antigen in a delivery device so that the vaccine can be administered to individuals
- Produce the vaccine in bulk
- Distribute the vaccine globally

The sum of all this required research and effort is much greater than that associated with other pharmaceutical products (including medications), which are not subject to such stringent production regulations. Vaccine development also requires significant resources and expertise in *process development*, or defining all steps necessary to make a product according to specific requirements, which is often not available at academic research centers.

Regulatory agencies such as the FDA provide guidance and oversight for the clinical development and manufacturing of vaccines that are split between research centers and pharmaceutical companies. Public health agencies such as the CDC become involved after licensure to monitor the epidemiology of the diseases prevented by the vaccines and make recommendations for the use of licensed vaccines in accordance with their findings. Increasingly, nongovernmental organizations are also becoming involved in vaccine development, primarily through funding specific initiatives or supporting partnerships to develop vaccines for diseases that affect mostly developing countries. A primary example is the Bill and Melinda Gates Foundation, which funds both the International AIDS Vaccine Initiative and the Malaria Vaccine Initiative. The relationship between all of these organizations is sometimes brokered by Program for Appropriate Technology in Health (PATH), which facilitates partnerships between companies to develop vaccine technologies that will work for developing countries. The many voices and players that populate the world of vaccine development have served to advance vaccine research, to standardize practices to ensure vaccine safety and efficacy, and, at times, to bureaucratize vaccine development.

How many vaccine manufacturers are there?

Including all companies that contribute to vaccine development and production, there are approximately 100 vaccine manufacturers globally. The vast majority are biotechnology or regional companies located in the United States, China, India, Japan, Korea, the European Union, and South America, but there are also some companies operating in Africa, Cuba, and the Middle East. These smaller companies may contribute a certain technology to a larger initiative or participate in development and distribution within a specific territory. Also, because these smaller companies are unlikely to have the infrastructure to scale-up or manufacture on a large scale, they are likely to license their work to a larger company.

Of the previously mentioned 100 manufacturers, only approximately 10 are large enough to participate in or independently conduct all aspects of vaccine development, from clinical research to manufacturing, distribution, and marketing. Of these 10, approximately half are actively invested in vaccine development. This list includes familiar names such as Merck, Pfizer, Sanofi, and GlaxoSmithKline. Each of these companies has an expansive vaccine development operation, and together they comprise nearly 90% of the global market share of vaccine manufacturing.

What actually happens in vaccine manufacturing?

Step 1: Generate the antigen(s)

This step differs by individual vaccine. First, manufacturers must produce the virus or bacteria and then either inactivate it (as with a live attenuated vaccine such as measles–mumps–rubella) or isolate the specific parts, or antigens, to be used in the vaccine. Viruses cannot live completely on their own; they need to grow on other cells. Thus, a manufacturing plant that makes vaccines is largely focused on making and maintaining cell cultures. For example, in the production of influenza vaccines, the influenza virus that is later attenuated or inactivated is first grown in an 11-day-old egg. The production of recombinant vaccines, in which genetic material is inserted into a different cell to make a certain protein, is another practice that requires ongoing maintenance of cell cultures.

Whatever the process required for antigen production, it must be tightly controlled to prevent contamination and to ensure that as much antigen as possible can be produced. Most manufacturers have a bank of cells that they use and reproduce to ensure consistency.

Step 2: Isolate and purify the antigens

Once antigens are produced, they are purified using some of the practices described in Chapter 1. This is followed by the addition of stabilizers or adjuvants that can extend the shelf life of a vaccine or enhance the immune response that the vaccine elicits. All vaccine components are placed in a single vial as a final formulation.

Step 3: Quality control

The final vaccine formulation undergoes several quality control steps to confirm its sterility, potency, and purity. If the formulation passes these tests, it is placed into sterile vials for final inspection and distribution. If the formulation does not pass the required quality control steps, the entire batch is discarded.

Vaccine manufacturing plants are expensive to build and maintain, mostly because of the complexity of vaccine production and the regulations that govern it. Vaccines may also require multiple plants to accommodate different aspects of the production process, necessitating several years of lead time before licensure to build a full-scale vaccine production plant. Thus, a company may have a facility for small-scale production early on and then move to commercial production capabilities.

What quality controls govern vaccine manufacturing?

Quality control safeguards are standard across every step of vaccine production, from process (or bulk manufacturing) to finishing. "Process" refers to antigen production and purification; "finishing" is the addition of stabilizing substances, vial filling, and packaging. Every substance used to make a vaccine must match very tight definitions to ensure that each has the properties promised and detailed in the approval and licensing stages of vaccine development. Every vaccine batch is tested to confirm its sterility and the presence of enough antigens to be effective. Vaccines are also evaluated for toxicity (in animals) before they are released. If anything during the process does not pass, vaccines are not released to the public. Adding to the complexity for manufacturers, vaccine requirements and regulations differ by country, so the same vaccine may require packaging in several different forms to meet the various requirements and distribution needs of its individual markets.

Who pays for vaccine development?

Funding comes from a range of sources. Basic research is generally supported by grants from federal agencies (e.g., the NIH) and is therefore supported by tax dollars. Other agencies, such as the FDA or the Department of Defense, may also provide research funds or include research activities in their own budgets. Foundations may also offer grants for vaccine research. Last, the private sector may also play a role: Some private investors may support vaccine manufacturers, especially smaller companies performing basic research. For larger pharmaceutical companies (e.g., the "big five" mentioned previously), profits from sales of existing vaccines are reinvested to support development of new vaccines; these investments generally represent approximately 18% of the companies' total profits. Approved vaccines are generally profitable because, unlike with medications, the production of generic vaccines is relatively rare—mostly because it is difficult for other would-be manufacturers to gain access to the specific technology needed for certain vaccines. In addition, new births—generally not in short supply—represent an ongoing market for vaccines.

This business model, however, does not always work well for developing countries. Although there may be a need, there may also be distribution challenges that demand additional resources. In addition, immunization programs in developing countries are not able to consistently pay for vaccines. Last, some diseases may affect only certain areas and consequently have a smaller market. Accordingly, pharmaceutical companies have less incentive for distribution globally. In the face of these challenges, there have been attempts to incentivize pharmaceutical companies into developing markets through strategies such as "advance market commitments." In these instances, the promise of profits from developed countries is leveraged to urge pharmaceutical companies to subsidize distribution in developing countries. Additional relief has recently come from emerging manufacturers in middle-income countries, which are stepping in to meet need in their own countries and, in some instances, globally. Examples include the Serum Institute in India, which produce measles, rubella, and diphtheria, tetanus, and pertussis (DTP) vaccines for more than 140 countries. Vaccine manufacturers in Brazil and China, which produce a massive amount of vaccines to support their own populations, are currently working on prequalification arrangements for export to other countries.

How much does vaccine development cost?

As vaccine technology has become more complex, the estimated cost of development for one vaccine has increased from $231 million in 1991 to $802 million in 2003 and $1 billion in 2010. These estimates include both post-licensure studies for approved vaccines and research and development activities that take place on failed products that do not pass early phase trials. A vaccine manufacturer may invest $100 million per year in vaccine development but only make one vaccine every 6–8 years.

How do manufacturers know how much vaccine to make?

Vaccine manufacturers estimate demand based on the size of the population that the vaccine targets, the strength of the scientific recommendations for its use, and the past performances of other similar vaccines. Initial supply may not keep up with demand, or it may be greater than demand. When the supply is greater than demand, the risk of wasting unused vaccines increases: All vaccines have an expiration date after which their effectiveness cannot be guaranteed.

Are there vaccine supply shortages?

Vaccine supply shortages happen fairly regularly, either due to underestimation of demand or due to production problems. If there is any issue fulfilling quality control measures, an entire batch of a vaccine may be wasted or thrown out. Especially for vaccines that are more complex to make, it can then take time to replace that batch, resulting in a shortage.

What happens when there are vaccine shortages?

Immunization program officials may recommend that health care providers administer one fewer dose in a vaccine series (remember that some vaccines require multiple doses) until the vaccine supply recovers. In other cases, a child will need to follow a catch-up schedule once the vaccine is available. There may also be an effort to prioritize vaccination to groups that are at highest risk for becoming infected or are suffering infection at a disproportionate rate.

4

VACCINE FINANCING
AND DISTRIBUTION

Making and manufacturing vaccines is only the first part of
the story in getting vaccines into public health programs and
health care facilities: Someone has to pay for them and facilitate their distribution. These practices and decisions can vary
significantly by region and country.

How are vaccines distributed once they are licensed?

Approval of a vaccine does not necessarily mean it will auto-
matically end up in clinics or pharmacies for distribution.
There must first be a distribution system in place to purchase
vaccines from manufacturers and distribute vaccines to clinics.
For this to happen, public health systems must decide whether
the vaccine should be added to their immunization program—
the schedule and roster of vaccines that are recommended as
standard for its population. In this process, similar to the steps
that inform vaccine development, policymakers consider the
burden of the disease that would be prevented by vaccination, along with vaccine cost and their ability to maintain an
adequate supply. Vaccines require certain storage and hand-
ling procedures to ensure that they remain stable and effective (refrigeration or cold chain, the latter of which can be very
difficult to maintain in resource-limited settings), and such
requirements are a necessary part of a national or local public

health body's decision as to whether to include a vaccine in its immunization program.

Some countries may not have the budget to add every newly developed vaccine. For example, most low-income countries use the whole cell diphtheria–tetanus–pertussis (DTP) vaccine, which was first introduced in 1948 and was used worldwide until the 1990s, when a new acellular version of the vaccine was introduced. The newer vaccine is better tolerated because it has fewer antigens, meaning that it is less likely to produce some of the side effects, such as high fever, that were seen with the first whole cell pertussis vaccine. Acellular pertussis vaccines are now used exclusively in the United States and several other countries. However, the newer vaccine is also more expensive to make and therefore costs more for recipients—too much for the budgets of many low-income countries, which continue to use DTP. The same is true with regard to measles vaccines. They are used in just about every country with an immunization program, but not every country uses the measles–mumps–rubella vaccine that is standard in the United States: Many use measles alone, or measles–rubella vaccines, due to cost differences.

Conversely, some vaccines used by the majority of the world's population are not used in the United States. This includes the bacille Calmette–Guérin (BCG) tuberculosis vaccine, which is given to infants worldwide to prevent severe tuberculosis infection in places where tuberculosis is *endemic*, or widespread (i.e., most of the world). Tuberculosis definitely occurs in the United States, but it is no longer endemic, and accordingly the country does not include this vaccine in its routine schedule.

Are there other vaccines used in some places but not others?

Vaccine programs vary across countries based on resources and the diseases that are endemic. All immunization programs generally include vaccines against measles, diphtheria, tetanus, pertussis, and polio. Most also include hepatitis

B, *Haemophilus influenzae* type b, and tuberculosis vaccines. Newer vaccines against pneumococcus and rotavirus, two of the most common causes of illness and death among children worldwide, are now available and also widely used in many national programs. However, due to their steep costs, these vaccines are being slowly incorporated into immunization programs in low- and middle-income countries.

On the other hand, some vaccines are very specific to a region and may be left off immunization programs elsewhere. These include vaccines for diseases such as yellow fever or Japanese encephalitis, which are a part of immunization programs in certain countries in which these diseases are common. In the United States, the standard meningococcal vaccine protects against four different types of meningococcus. Other countries, such as many in the European Union, use a meningococcal vaccine against only one or two types of the disease. These different practices reflect the differences in incidence of disease and strain distribution across regions and countries.

How much do vaccines actually cost for immunization programs?

The retail prices of vaccines vary widely and reflect the costs of their development, production, and distribution. Some vaccines are easier to make than others, so the more complex the vaccine, the more expensive it is. End-user costs can range from less than $1 per individual vaccine (as with the measles–mumps–rubella vaccine) to $160 per dose (for the human papillomavirus vaccine). Costs may also depend on who is doing the negotiating: Vaccine companies may consider the value of a vaccine for a given society or country along with the ability to purchase vaccine and then reduce the price accordingly.

In addition to the cost of the actual vaccine, costs associated with vaccine administration increase the overall expense of vaccine programs. Generally, this is due to requirements for vaccine storage (i.e., refrigeration) or administrative activities such as medical record-keeping and reporting. Registry systems for vaccinations are common, and they require the ongoing maintenance and transmittal of immunization records. Increasingly, this is done through electronic medical records, which in the United States were a major component of the Affordable Care Act that included requirements for reporting vaccine doses to immunization registries. Although there are benefits to reporting immunization rates, setting up these electronic systems requires significant resources. All of these factors have resulted in increasing costs and, at times, financial barriers to the administration of vaccines in developed and developing countries, even to groups for whom a vaccine is recommended for routine use.

How large is the vaccine market?

Market size is another factor that is largely dependent on uptake by vaccine programs across public health. A vaccine can go through all the steps for licensure and gain approval for use from the US Food and Drug Administration, but if there is no recommendation to use the vaccine, it most likely will not be covered by insurance and will not likely be recommended by providers. Without either of these features, the vaccine is not likely to be used, meaning there is no market for it.

Vaccines that are adopted by vaccine programs represent a sizable revenue stream for manufacturers (albeit at a significant launch cost, as detailed elsewhere). Vaccines produce an estimated global market revenue of $25 billion for vaccine companies, with 85% going to the top five Western manufacturers. Despite this significant share of the global revenue, these manufacturers have a comparatively small market share, providing only 52% of vaccine doses worldwide.

Who decides which vaccine should be distributed?

As discussed previously, vaccine distribution and financing vary by country and are mostly dictated by national vaccine policies. In the United States, no one group drives decision-making about vaccine development and distribution. Early in vaccine history, new vaccines were developed by individual scientists, or groups of scientists, from universities or foundations, and pharmaceutical companies would then take new vaccines forward to production and distribution. In these early days, vaccines were not a part of national public health policy: They were available, but access was not necessarily guaranteed. They were instead utilized in specific situations of need, such as a disease outbreak or among military recruits residing in close quarters.

In the United States, widespread distribution of vaccines did not occur until federal policy increased funding for vaccine procurement and development and strengthened school entry requirements. In 1961, President John F. Kennedy passed the Vaccine Appropriations Act, which established the first semblance of a national immunization program. The act subsidized purchase of measles and polio vaccines by states, broadening access and establishing vaccination as a right rather than an ad hoc tool. Nonetheless, access to vaccines remained uneven, with significant socioeconomic disparities between low-income children and those in other income strata.

To spark additional vaccine development, the US National Institutes of Health established the Vaccine Development Board in 1965 to provide grants for vaccine research. At the same time, President Lyndon B. Johnson approved funding to provide federal grants for immunization as part of an initiative to increase life expectancy. Yet, while the national immunization program expanded, there was little consistency: Funding commitments for research changed with administrations, as they do today. There was also little consistency in vaccination laws across states in terms of requirements or their enforcement, leading to a wide range in rates across communities and ongoing outbreaks. In 1977, under the Carter Administration, the national immunization program received a significant push with increased funding for vaccine grants and a campaign to encourage states to strengthen school entry immunization requirements. These measures coincided with (or perhaps fueled) a swell in public uptake of vaccines. By the end of 1979, immunization rates were up 90% among schoolchildren, and because immunizations were an established part of the US health care system, there was a reliable market for ongoing vaccine distribution and development.

The 1980s brought the establishment of the National Vaccine Advisory Committee (NVAC), an advisory group responsible for setting priorities for the national immunization program.

What is the National Vaccine Advisory Committee?

NVAC is a federal advisory commission charged with evaluating vaccine policy in the United States and making recommendations to strengthen the US immunization program. It sits within the National Vaccine Program Office in the Department of Health and Human Services. Its charge targets four domains: (1) ensure availability of an adequate supply of safe and effective vaccines, (2) identify research priorities to support vaccine safety and effectiveness, (3) advise the Assistant Secretary of Health on implementation of the National Vaccine Plan, and (4) identify opportunities for governmental and nongovernmental cooperation.

The committee comprises 17 voting members (14 public members that include health care providers, public health practitioners, and members of immunization-related organizations; 2 vaccine researchers or manufacturers; and 1 committee chair). The committee may also include ex officio and liaison members from different federal agencies, and it may also spin off to form working groups to address specific topics (e.g., immunizations for pregnant women and vaccine hesitancy). These working groups include committee members as well as outside individuals who may have expertise on a given topic.

How does the National Vaccine Advisory Committee impact vaccine policy?

Recommendations from NVAC have resulted in policy changes. In 1991, the committee issued a report about measles in the face of a measles epidemic that cited significant barriers to ensuring high measles vaccine coverage, including costs and adequate research to measure the determinants of immunization coverage. The report influenced the establishment of the Vaccines for Children (VFC) program, which today provides vaccines free of charge to publicly insured, uninsured and underinsured children younger than age 18 years, as well as the National Immunization Survey, through which immunization rates are monitored annually. Both of these programs are key components of our current immunization system. Relatively recently, NVAC has issued recommendations and reports about using immunization registries, recommendations for vaccinating pregnant women, and vaccine confidence. NVAC has also commissioned the Institute of Medicine (now the National Academy of Medicine), an independent public policy research group, to develop a decision support tool to help guide prioritization for vaccine development. The tool, called SMART Vaccines, can be applied to any setting and uses much of the same information reviewed in Chapter 3: characteristics of the population, disease burden, characteristics of the vaccine, and information related to benefits and costs.

What is the National Vaccine Plan?

The National Vaccine Plan was established by the National Vaccine Program Office in 2010 to provide a way to lay out a multifaceted strategy to support the immunization program in the United States and internationally. The plan focuses on the following five main areas: the development of new and better vaccines, improved communication about vaccines, enhancement of the vaccine safety infrastructure, a stable and accessible supply of recommended vaccines, and improved capacity of immunization programs in other countries. This final charge is a product of globalization, through which vaccine-preventable diseases can easily be imported into the United States through travel or immigration. Immunization rates worldwide can therefore affect what Americans may be exposed to when traveling or what returning Americans or non-American visitors may bring with them when they enter the United States.

Similar to the National Vaccine Plan in the United States, there is also a Global Vaccine Action Plan, which was endorsed by the World Health Assembly in 2012 as a part of the Decade of Vaccines.

What are the Decade of Vaccines and the Global Vaccine Action Plan?

The Decade of Vaccines Collaboration was launched in 2010 by a group of nongovernmental organizations (including the Gates Foundation, United Nations Initiative for Children and Families, and the World Health Organization (WHO)) and the US National Institutes of Health, in addition to partners from national immunization programs, the general public, and vaccine manufacturers, to increase equitable access to vaccines worldwide and prevent death from vaccine-preventable diseases. The centerpiece of the collaboration was the Global Vaccine Action Plan, which lays out goals to be achieved by 2020: the introduction of new or underutilized vaccines in at least 80 low- and middle-income countries, the expansion of immunization services to achieve at least 90% national vaccination coverage rates, global polio eradication, and significant reductions in childhood mortality.

To pursue these goals, the Collaboration employed a set of six strategies:

1. Encourage all countries to make immunization and evidence-based decisions a priority

2. Educate community members about the value of vaccines, encouraging members to demand immunization as a right and responsibility
3. Promote equitable distribution of immunization benefits
4. Elevate immunization systems as an integral component to a strong health system
5. Facilitate governments' sustainable access to vaccine funding, supply, and new technologies
6. Support research that maximizes the benefits of immunization

Enacting these strategies has been largely accomplished through infrastructure and resources provided by WHO, with supplemental support from partnerships with collaborative organizations that help support vaccine financing and service delivery. The Gates Foundation, for example, pledged $10 billion to the Decade of Vaccines when it was first established in 2010.

Once a vaccine is added to an immunization program, how does it get to the people who need it?

In the United States, vaccines are typically delivered in a clinic, where individuals schedule an appointment to see a health care provider. Vaccines are part of a larger health maintenance visit in which patients may receive a physical exam, height and weight monitoring, and counseling on a range of health topics. In other settings, vaccines are given in clinics, but this may not be tied to a visit with a pediatrician, internist, or other health care practitioner. Instead, specific immunization days are hosted by a health care facility, and individuals come solely to receive vaccines for themselves or their children.

When access to health care services is limited, vaccine clinics may also be set up in other community sites. In some instances, especially for immunization campaigns that are trying to reach everyone in a community, vaccines may be distributed door to door. Alternative strategies are also used for groups that are less likely to have regular health care contact. For example, adolescents and adults are less likely to go to a clinic for regular health care services; this is true in both developed and developing countries. Thus, immunization programs may consider vaccine delivery in alternative locations such as schools or pharmacies.

What is required to be able to deliver vaccines in a clinic or community setting?

There are a few important requirements for any setting in which vaccines are administered. First, vaccines are highly temperature sensitive, so storage is a key consideration from the moment a vaccine leaves the manufacturer. Because vaccines need to be refrigerated or frozen, their transport and storage require some kind of "cold chain" that keeps vaccines at a certain temperature until the time of administration. Refrigerators and freezers in vaccine storage and transportation devices must be monitored very closely to ensure that a certain temperature range is maintained. If a vaccine is not stored properly, it may not work as well.

Needless to say, maintaining a cold chain is particularly challenging in warm climates, especially in resource-limited settings in which power sources may not be reliable and transport options are more limited. Maintaining a cold chain is therefore a major part of immunization program management in low- and middle-income countries, particularly the development of new strategies to make cold chains easier to maintain. It is also a significant part of program management in developed countries, including the United States.

Of course, vaccine administration also requires personnel who have been trained to give vaccines. Most vaccines are delivered into muscle or just under the skin, and technique is important to ensure that the vaccine is delivered properly and to prevent injuries related to injection. In most cases, the individuals who deliver vaccines have a background in nursing, and in some places, including the United States, pharmacists may also deliver them.

How are vaccines purchased by health care facilities?

How vaccines get to the site of administration depends on whether vaccines are financed through a public or a private system. In simple terms, when vaccines are part of the public health system, they are purchased by the government or health agency in the given country and then distributed to health care facilities. In a private system, health care facilities purchase vaccines and then charge individuals (or, more likely, individuals' insurance) for administration.

In the United States and many other countries, there is a mixed public and private system that relies on insurance coverage. Generally, insurance, whether public or private, covers vaccines that have been recommended for *routine use*. Routine use means that everyone in a certain group (i.e., age cohort) should receive that particular vaccine. For privately insured patients, providers will purchase vaccine directly from manufacturers or distribution centers and then bill patients' insurance plans for both the vaccine and administration costs. However, the amount of coverage may vary. Some private plans cover most, but not all, recommended vaccines, or they may cover the cost of the vaccine but not administration costs. Others cover vaccines up to a certain amount. If a private insurance plan does not cover the purchase or administration of one or more vaccines, a child is considered "underinsured" and may seek to receive vaccines through a public source such as the federal VFC program.

How are vaccines purchased through public insurance?

There are three primary mechanisms through which vaccines are purchased on the public (i.e., federally funded) side of the US health care system: the VFC program, the Title 317 federal grant program to states, and individual states' discretionary funds. As the immunization program in the United States grew during the 1970s and 1980s, significant disparities emerged between insured and uninsured children, the latter of whom were likely to go unvaccinated unless their parents paid out of pocket. To address this gap, the US Department of Health and Human Services established the VFC program in 1994 to ensure the provision of vaccines for uninsured, publicly insured (i.e., eligible for Medicaid), and American Indian/Alaska Native children 18 years of age or younger. The program purchases vaccines from vaccine manufacturers and then distributes them to providers who provide care to VFC-eligible children via health departments. The vaccine is provided without charge to the provider or child. However, the VFC program does not cover any charges associated with giving the vaccine (i.e., supplies or vaccine storage costs). Although the vaccine itself is free, providers may charge an administration fee but cannot refuse vaccination if a family cannot pay. Underinsured children can also receive VFC program vaccines if they receive care at certain sites, a federally qualified health center, or a rural health center.

For individuals older than age 18 years or children who are not eligible for the VFC program but whose insurance does not cover certain vaccines, Title 317 funds may be used. However, in contrast to VFC, this program is not an entitlement—that is, there is no guarantee of funds to purchase vaccines for all individuals who may be eligible for the program. Title 317 is a discretionary fund with a budget that fluctuates every year, and accordingly states may not have enough funding each year to purchase vaccines for everyone who may be eligible for the program. As a result, coverage varies quite significantly by state. To supplement Title 317, states therefore may use discretionary funds to purchase vaccines for non-VFC eligible children. In recent years, it has been difficult for states to maintain enough funds to keep up with the rising costs of an expanding immunization program.

How do people without insurance or who do not qualify for publicly funded programs access vaccines?

If a patient is not insured and does not qualify for a publicly funded program that supplies vaccines, that individual would have to pay for the vaccine himself or herself; this may also be the case for vaccines that are not covered by insurance. In general, vaccines covered by insurance programs include those that are routinely recommended for children or adults (these recommendations are discussed in Chapter 6). Health insurance benefits vary widely, but most do cover regularly utilized health care interventions and services. With the passage of the Affordable Care Act in 2010, health plans are required to cover 10 essential benefits, including preventive services such as immunizations. However, for vaccines that are only given in special circumstances, such as those needed for travel, there is often no insurance coverage. In these cases, the vaccine must be paid for by the individual at the time of administration.

Who purchases most of the vaccines in the United States?

The public sector purchases just over half of all vaccines for children in the United States, but most vaccines are still given in private physician offices. This is because most private physicians can give both publicly and privately purchased vaccines—the source of the vaccines a provider gives depends on the insurance coverage and VFC eligibility of the patient he or she is seeing. Thus, if a provider is seeing a publicly insured patient who qualifies for VFC, the provider can use only VFC vaccine. If the provider is seeing a patient who is not VFC eligible, the provider can use only privately purchased vaccine. On rare occasions (and with approval from the VFC program), a provider may borrow a private stock vaccine for a

VFC-eligible patient but the vaccine dose needs to be replaced. Generally, publicly and privately covered vaccines are similar, particularly for vaccines routinely recommended for children. However, there may some differences in the specific brands covered by the VFC program and private insurers.

Who sets priorities for vaccine distribution in non-US countries?

For the most part, every country has its own national immunization program that governs vaccine policy based on the burden of disease within the country and the costs associated with purchase and distribution. For low- and middle-income countries, vaccine policy is largely dictated by WHO, which provides guidance and infrastructure for vaccine development, regulatory review, vaccine distribution, immunization recommendations, and disease surveillance. The cornerstone of WHO immunization activities is the Expanded Program on Immunization (EPI).

What is the Expanded Program on Immunization?

EPI was established in 1974 to support the development of national immunization programs in countries throughout the world. EPI was built on momentum from the global eradication of smallpox, which was achieved with the benefit of global infrastructure to support smallpox vaccine delivery.

EPI makes recommendations to governments related to which vaccines will have the largest impact on reducing childhood illness and death. When the program was first established, it recommended vaccines against diphtheria, tetanus, pertussis, measles, and polio; subsequently, its recommendation expanded to include hepatitis B, *Haemophilus influenzae* b, and, for some countries, yellow fever. The program has continued to incorporate new vaccines to guide national immunization programs, but more important, it also provides resources to help national programs adopt recommendations. The goal of EPI is universal immunization for all children in every country, which is a difficult task in light of the vast differences in resources across countries.

How does the World Health Organization support other countries?

WHO has myriad resources to increase implementation of EPI and support national immunization programs. One such mechanism is the National Immunization Technical Advisory Groups—country-specific groups that advise policymakers and immunization program managers. Most developed and some developing countries have one of these groups, which can share resources from the WHO, including EPI. This might include anything from guidance regarding new vaccines to tools for financing immunizations. A WHO program called Vaccine Product, Price, and Procurement is employed to support accurate and reliable product and price information for vaccines in areas where sustainability is a concern, and WHO can supplement it with partnerships to other organizations that can help support vaccine supply and financing.

WHO's implementation strategies are summarized in a comprehensive publication titled *Global Routine Immunization Strategies and Practice*, which serves as a sort of manual for guiding activities of immunization programs. Its recommendations are largely centered on building infrastructure and governance: building a national team, targeting under- and unvaccinated populations, utilizing coherent planning, ensuring adequate funding, investing in vaccinators, updating vaccine supply chain and information systems, expanding routine schedules, and sharing responsibility for immunization delivery. WHO can provide this guidance, but it is not always the lone bearer of financial burdens associated with implementation.

How does vaccine financing happen in non-US countries, including low- to middle-income countries?

For the purchase of vaccines, some countries have a public–private insurance dichotomy similar to that in the United States; in others, almost all vaccines are distributed through the public health system, meaning that vaccines are purchased using government funds. In cases of bulk purchasing by governments, these agencies are often able to negotiate a lower price per vaccine and then distribute the vaccines to clinics for administration. In these settings, immunization programs are largely dependent on the availability of government funds as well as political will to prioritize immunization programs. Because vaccine-purchasing decisions may affect the availability of resources for other public health activities, some countries consider cost-effectiveness and systematically weigh the potential benefits of introducing a certain vaccine against the cost of introduction.

How are vaccines made more accessible to lower income countries?

Low- to middle-income countries may need to forgo certain vaccines due to budget constraints and infrastructure limitations, even if the vaccines would be highly impactful. Pneumococcal, rotavirus, and human papillomavirus vaccines are examples of vaccines that are newer and more expensive and thus less common in countries with fewer resources. There are different mechanisms by which countries can work to procure vaccines at lower cost. One particularly successful and impactful program is the Global Alliance for Vaccines and Immunizations (GAVI), which stands as arguably the global leader in financing vaccines through public–private partnership.

GAVI was founded in Switzerland in 2000 to increase access to immunizations and build capacity for sustained investment in immunization programs—beyond the core six vaccines distributed through EPI and with deeper penetration in resource-limited areas. Countries that meet certain criteria (e.g., gross annual income less than $1,580 per capita) can apply for support from GAVI, which will in turn provide funding to purchase vaccines during a given period of time. The participating nation must commit to contributing a small amount to the financing of vaccines, with a broader goal of increasing infrastructure development and establishing a mechanism to increase co-financing contributions and build toward full self-financing.

GAVI began with a $750 million pledge from the Gates Foundation, and since then it has leveraged funds from developed countries and foundations to negotiate lower prices on vaccine purchases across territories—making vaccines more affordable and accessible while also helping vaccine manufacturers find a footing in emerging markets and liaising with service organizations to help with vaccine delivery. Countries that receive support from GAVI are able to take the lead in applying funds to their immunization programs, and they can apply for additional support to introduce any of the 10 GAVI-supported vaccines into a national immunization program (or to implement an immunization campaign to increase rates). GAVI-supported vaccines include those associated with the most childhood illness and death worldwide.

In 2015, 73 countries received GAVI support, and 4 countries were able to transition out of support to independently finance and implement their immunization programs. What is the impact? Between 2010 and 2015, an additional 277 million children received a GAVI-supported vaccine, helping to prevent an estimated 4 million deaths.

Other programs have also supported vaccine distribution in resource-limited settings, including the Fund for Vaccine Procurement, which was established by the Pan-American Heath Organization to help procure vaccines as well as cold chain supplies for Latin American countries. This program has also utilized bulk purchasing to help provide a steady supply of vaccines. The Program for Appropriate Technology in Health (PATH) is another global nonprofit organization that helps support the development of vaccines against diseases such as malaria, in addition to new vaccine technologies that make it easier to safely store and deliver vaccines.

5

VACCINE SAFETY

"Are vaccines safe?" has become one of the most hotly contested and politically charged questions in contemporary culture, fueled in no small part by voracious online debates, peer-to-peer influence, and source information of varying degrees of quality and accuracy. Along with questions related to possible side effects, the vaccine schedule has also come under question among parents, with some now choosing to deviate from the timing recommended by pediatricians for vaccinating children.

Vaccines have an excellent safety profile and are governed by a rigorous set of federal regulations, but no medication or intervention is 100% risk-free. This chapter reviews reactions that can occur after vaccination and also the other safety concerns for which well-established evidence does not support an association. Last, this chapter describes the vaccine safety program in the United States to highlight the many mechanisms through which safety is monitored.

What is a vaccine adverse event?

A *vaccine adverse event* is the appearance of any symptom after receiving a vaccine. When the symptom or health problem can be causally traced back to the administration of a vaccine, the symptom is a vaccine side effect. An example is fever: Because vaccines induce an immune response as a way of prompting the body to produce antibodies, the immune response may bring about an increase in body temperature. This fever is considered a vaccine side effect because it can be uncomfortable and may also cause anxiety; it also would not have occurred had the individual not received the vaccine.

However, not all new symptoms that develop after receiving a vaccine are a result of the vaccination. It is easy to attribute anything that occurs soon after receiving a vaccine to vaccination, but timing does not always mean causation.

How can one determine whether an adverse event is really caused by a vaccine?

Monitoring vaccine recipients for adverse events is a major part of vaccine development. Even before a vaccine is first tested in people, the potential for adverse events is considered. When trials in people begin, scientists measure not only how well the vaccine works but also how well the vaccine is tolerated. This is measured by comparing how many adverse events occur among those who receive the vaccine (the experimental group) against how many occur in those who do not receive the vaccine (the placebo, or control, group). During these studies, participants in both groups are asked to report any illness or symptom they experience within a certain time period after receiving the vaccine or the placebo. If there is no difference in the frequency of reported symptoms in the experimental and placebo groups, it means there is no indication that the symptom is due to vaccination; it is just as likely to occur without vaccination. If the reported symptoms occur more frequently in the vaccinated group than in the placebo group, it suggests the symptom may be associated with vaccination. These findings are included in the reports reviewed by the US Food and Drug Administration (FDA) before a vaccine is approved, and all of the reported events—even those that are not necessarily associated with vaccination—are listed in the package insert that accompanies all vaccines and medications that are approved by the FDA.

In attempting to establish possible causation between a vaccine and an event, a few additional criteria are employed to determine whether an adverse event is truly vaccine-related. One of them is considering whether it is biologically possible for an event to be associated with a vaccine. In other words, there must be a way to explain how receiving the vaccine in question could result in the reported symptom.

How is safety monitored after a vaccine is licensed?

Monitoring for safety events does not stop after licensure. The 2007 Food and Drug Administration Act mandates that the FDA develop a safety surveillance program for ongoing monitoring of all vaccines, and any company that has submitted an application for licensure must also provide a plan to conduct ongoing safety surveillance studies. These ongoing surveillance activities are important because some outcomes may be so rare that they would not be detected during the prelicensure studies.

In the United States, multiple systems function for vaccine safety surveillance. One is the Vaccine Adverse Events Reporting System (VAERS), which was established by the Centers for Disease Control and Prevention (CDC) and the FDA in 1986 as a part of the National Vaccine Injury Compensation Program to perform surveillance for safety events. Anytime a new symptom occurs within a certain time period after receipt of any vaccine, it can be reported to the system, which is regularly monitored by medical officers from the FDA and the CDC. Whenever the officers note a signal, or multiple reports of a symptom following a certain vaccine, an investigation is initiated to determine whether the connection between receiving a particular vaccine and developing the new symptom is causal. In other words, investigators test whether the symptom is more likely to occur among people who just received the vaccine than among people who have not received the vaccine.

It is important to note that VAERS is a *passive surveillance system*, meaning it captures only events reported by people who have experienced a symptom that they think may be related to a vaccine. This means the system may not capture all potential adverse events, and it may also capture events that are not related to vaccination. In addition, because it only tallies events among people who have just been vaccinated, it lacks a comparison (control) group of people who have not received the vaccine to measure whether the event would be as likely to occur without vaccination. For these reasons, VAERS as a stand-alone system is not suited to independently confirm whether an adverse event is associated with a vaccine; it is a screening tool.

Who can report to VAERS?

Events can be reported by health care providers, vaccine recipients (or their guardians), or vaccine manufacturers. There is a reporting mandate for health care providers and vaccine manufacturers as part of the National Vaccine Injury Compensation Program (described later) that requires reporting for (1) any adverse event that has been listed by the vaccine manufacturer as a contraindication for receiving additional doses of the vaccine and (2) any adverse event that is listed in the VAERS table and develops within a certain time period after vaccination. The VAERS table includes specific adverse events that have been previously associated with a licensed vaccine from vaccine safety studies. An example is anaphylaxis or a severe allergic reaction, which can occur if someone has an allergy to a vaccine component. However, this mandate does not prevent reporting of other symptoms that are not included in the table.

Reports can be submitted online, by fax, or by mail using a form that requests several pieces of information about the event. However, completion of all items is not a requirement, nor is there a way to validate information at the time of submission. The form was updated in 2014 to improve ease of use and include more information about health status and patient characteristics that can help medical officers in their initial review.

How often are reports submitted to VAERS?

Approximately 30,000 reports are submitted to VAERS each year, of which the vast majority (87–90%) are mild, self-resolving events such as fever and swelling and pain around the vaccine's injection site. To put that figure into context, more than 10 million vaccine doses are delivered to children and 145 million doses of influenza vaccine are distributed across all age groups each year.

What happens when VAERS finds a signal?

The occurrence of multiple, similar symptoms or a report of a serious adverse event will prompt medical officers to take a closer look. For some cases, medical officers may contact the health care provider and patient to obtain more information about symptoms, timing, and medical history; there may also be additional follow-up over time to monitor for recovery. If there is concern that these reports could signal a new or emerging cluster of vaccine-related adverse events, this may prompt further investigation through the next major arm of the vaccine safety system, *active surveillance networks*. For example, the increased risk of intussusception associated with the first rotavirus vaccine (called Rotashield) in 1998 was first identified through reports to VAERS. When investigators noticed an increase in reported cases among infants, especially infants who would otherwise not be likely to develop intussusception, the CDC recommended suspending use of Rotashield. Two large studies ensued, each using active surveillance networks to evaluate whether the vaccine was associated with some cases of intussusception.

What are active surveillance networks?

Active surveillance refers to medical investigators' active monitoring for a specific condition or outcome in a population (as opposed to collecting reports of conditions or outcomes, which, as discussed previously, is *passive*). Active surveillance is a more robust method for studying vaccine-related adverse events because it allows capturing of all the events, such as fever, in a given population. Experts can then compare how frequently the symptom occurs between people who were and were not vaccinated within a certain time period. This allows for what is called *signal confirmation*.

Three active surveillance networks help perform studies to evaluate vaccine safety in the United States. The first is called the Vaccine Safety Datalink (VSD), which is a partnership between the CDC and nine different managed-care organizations throughout several states (e.g., Kaiser Permanente). The network comprises a patient population of 9 million children and adults, and it draws data from electronic medical records weekly to monitor for incidents that occur with recently vaccinated individuals. The network also has a built-in control group, which allows investigators to compare children who just received a certain vaccine to children who had a health care visit on the same day but did not receive a vaccine.

The second active surveillance network is the Clinical Immunization Safety Assessment Network (CISA), a network of seven academic medical centers connected by the CDC with the overall goal of pooling research to identify and manage vaccine-related adverse events. This network performs studies to identify whether certain people may be at higher risk for serious vaccine-related adverse events and to inform which contraindications or precautions should accompany the administration of a vaccine.

Third, the FDA hosts the Post-Licensure Rapid Immunization Safety Monitoring Program (PRISM), which was first established in 2009 to evaluate the safety of the 2009 H1N1 pandemic influenza vaccine. The system links electronic health record data with data from immunization registries, providing a means to evaluate a large, diverse patient population (nearly 40 million individuals from nine state immunization registries). It has therefore continued as a safety surveillance network even after the end of the H1N1 pandemic.

Several other vaccine safety networks and registries monitor specific populations (including people who have received specific vaccines). For example, the Vaccines and Medications in Pregnancy Surveillance System was established in 2009 to monitor the safety of vaccines and medication use during pregnancy. Studies to date have evaluated influenza and pertussis vaccines that are recommended for pregnant women.

What is the difference between the information provided by VAERS and that provided by these other active surveillance networks?

Information provided by VAERS tells officials about any symptom an individual develops after receiving a vaccine. Information provided by VSD, CISA, PRISMA, and other active surveillance networks tells officials whether specific symptoms are more or less likely to occur in people who were recently vaccinated compared to those who had not been vaccinated. This kind of information can help determine whether an adverse event is truly associated with a given vaccine.

What kind of reactions can occur after vaccination?

Reactions are classified as mild, moderate, or serious. Mild reactions such as fever and soreness/swelling at the injection site are the most commonly reported adverse events. These do not necessarily require medical care, and they generally self-resolve within 2 or 3 days.

Moderate to serious adverse events may last longer and accordingly may require medical intervention. These are much less common and include the following:

1. Fainting (syncope) has been associated with the receipt of vaccines by some adolescents and adults. It is caused by the body's *vasovagal response,* in which pain or stress cause heart rate and blood pressure to drop suddenly. (These types of responses can occur in any instance of stress, not just with vaccines.) Because fainting is a known potential adverse event, many practitioners will ask adolescent patients to remain seated for 15 minutes after receiving any vaccine.

2. Seizure associated with fever (febrile seizure) occurs when a child younger than age 5 years has a fever and has no other underlying condition that would cause a seizure (e.g., epilepsy). Approximately 1 in 20 children will have a febrile seizure at some point during childhood, often due to a fever from an infection. Febrile seizures are distressing but generally resolve on their own and do not reoccur; they also do not lead to the development of a seizure disorder. Because vaccination can cause a fever, the risk of a febrile seizure can also increase after receiving certain vaccines. This has been observed with measles, mumps, and rubella (MMR) vaccines, which were found to cause an additional one febrile seizure for every 10,000 vaccines administered to young children (compared to normal rates of febrile seizures). Patients who receive more than one vaccine at the same time may also have a modestly higher risk of febrile seizure, particularly when combining influenza vaccines with pneumococcal vaccines or the diphtheria–tetanus–acellular pertussis (DTaP) vaccine. A 2016 study that evaluated several years of data from the VSD found that these

combinations produced approximately three more febrile seizures per 100,000 vaccine administrations compared to receiving any of these vaccines separately. There is no indication that febrile seizures related to vaccination are more or less severe than commonplace febrile seizures related to fever from infection. In some cases, vaccination may reduce the risk of a febrile seizure in the course of a child's life because vaccines prevent fever-inducing infections; this was observed in two large studies that examined febrile seizures after rotavirus vaccination.

3. Shoulder injury related to vaccine administration (SIRVA) is an injury to the nerves lining the muscles in the shoulder, leading to prolonged pain and limited range of motion. SIRVA diminishes over time but can limit activity until it does diminish. It is important to note that this type of adverse event is related to how the vaccine is administered, not the vaccine itself; it can therefore happen after administration of any vaccine delivered in the shoulder.

4. Anaphylaxis is a severe allergic reaction that can occur if a person is allergic to a vaccine component. This occurs very rarely—as stated previously, one or two times for every 1 million doses of a vaccine given.

Individual vaccines are constantly monitored for new or common reactions, and the findings of these studies are summarized at https://www.cdc.gov/vaccines/vac-gen/side-effects.htm.

How often do adverse events really occur?

The frequency of adverse events can be considered in terms of the number of reports to a system such as VAERS. Again, however, there are events that occur within a certain time period after receiving a vaccine that are not necessarily caused by the vaccines. Thus, for known adverse events, such as fever or seizures with fever, it is more accurate to measure a rate—or an estimated number of events among a certain number of vaccinated people. Active surveillance data for specific events indicate that fever and local arm swelling can occur anywhere from 1 in 100 to 1 in 30 children and adolescents, depending on the vaccine. Moderate to severe events occur far less frequently— one time for every 10,000 doses for febrile seizures and one or two times for every 1 million doses for anaphylaxis.

Is Guillain–Barré syndrome associated with vaccines?

Guillain–Barré syndrome (GBS) is a rare neurologic condition that typically occurs after a person has had an infection (usually either influenza or certain strains of gastroenteritis, an illness associated with vomiting and diarrhea). A person with GBS creates antibodies that attack parts of the nervous system, causing muscle weakness in the limbs and in parts of the body associated with breathing and swallowing. Cases of GBS have also been reported after the receipt of certain vaccines, particularly influenza vaccines. The relationship between the two is extraordinarily difficult to study, mostly because GBS occurs very rarely (only one case per 1 million individuals, with or without vaccination). An increased risk for GBS was identified in association with the 1976 swine flu vaccine, although some question the association due to biased reporting and an imprecise case definition for GBS at that time. In any event, subsequent studies have not found an association between GBS and seasonal influenza vaccines since 1976. GBS has not occurred any more frequently among those who have received a vaccine compared to those who have not received a vaccine. However, because having a history of GBS can increase the likelihood of developing another episode of GBS later, most doctors use caution in administering influenza vaccines to people who previously had GBS within 6 weeks of an influenza vaccine.

What are contraindications to vaccination?

Vaccines are *contraindicated*—not recommended—in persons who, by virtue of their medical history, are at greater risk of experiencing an adverse event. The most common grounds for contraindication is a weakened immune system, which is known as immunodeficiency or immunocompromise. A weakened immune system can be a secondary symptom of an illness or, as with chemotherapy, a side effect of treatment for an illness. Whatever the cause or source, people with immunocompromising conditions are contraindicated for receipt of live attenuated vaccines (vaccines made of weakened viruses or bacteria) due to the potential risk of developing an infection from the weakened strain. A history of severe allergic reaction to a vaccine ingredient is also a contraindication to receiving that specific vaccine.

What are precautions?

In the context of vaccines, a *precaution* is any condition that may cause the vaccine to work less fully or optimally and accordingly may be grounds to delay administering the vaccine. A general precaution for vaccines is illness (with or without fever), which if present at the time of vaccination could cause an insufficient reaction by the already active immune system. (This is why physicians generally ask how patients are feeling before administering any vaccines.) A mild illness such as the common cold is not a precaution.

Some vaccines may also come with specific precautions, which are meant to minimize risk of an adverse event in certain individuals. For example, having a seizure disorder that is not well controlled is a precaution for people receiving pertussis (whooping cough)-containing vaccines, which in rare instances have been shown to activate seizures with or without fever in a small number of patients. In these instances, receiving a dose of a pertussis-containing vaccine may be delayed until the seizure disorder has stabilized; in more extreme cases in which the seizure disorder cannot be controlled, the pertussis vaccination might be delayed indefinitely. Delaying vaccination would likely be revisited in the event of a pertussis outbreak because the likelihood of an unvaccinated person contracting pertussis is far greater (and potentially more serious) than a seizure episode.

Another important precaution for some live attenuated (weakened virus) vaccines is the receipt of products that contain antibodies—in particular, blood products such as intravenous immunoglobulin (IVIG) that are used to treat autoimmune disorders. IVIG is a blood product that contains antibodies pooled from other people, and the antibodies from the blood product can bind to the virus in live attenuated vaccines or to the antigens in inactivated vaccines. In either case, it renders most of these vaccines ineffective.

Can a person be vaccinated if he or she is on an antibiotic?

Being on an antibiotic is not a precaution or contraindication to vaccination. Antibiotics kill living and reproducing bacteria. They have no effect on a virus, including live attenuated viruses. Other vaccines are made from a few proteins or antigens from bacteria, and an antibiotic would have no activity against these proteins. The exception is taking a medicine that can treat a virus, such as oseltamivir for influenza or acyclovir for herpes virus or varicella. Taking these medications soon after receiving a varicella or live virus influenza vaccine will make these vaccines less effective.

If a person is immunocompromised because of chemotherapy or an organ transplant, can he or she receive any vaccines?

In general, immunocompromised individuals are advised to avoid live attenuated vaccines while receiving chemotherapy or undergoing transplant. Inactivated vaccines could be given safely, meaning there is no risk of developing infection, but they are not likely to be effective because immunocompromised individuals do not have the immune strength to develop immunity after vaccination. However, vaccines are safe and perform well after immunosuppressive medications are stopped and the immune system has a chance to recover. This can take several weeks to months depending on the type of immunosuppressive medication and the individual's condition overall. Because being immunocompromised also places people at greater risk of becoming very sick from vaccine-preventable diseases, people who know that they will be receiving a transplant or starting chemotherapy should receive recommended vaccines in advance so that they will have some protection during and after treatment.

If a person was vaccinated before starting chemotherapy, will the effect of the vaccine last?

This depends on the type of chemotherapy. Some medications are so immunosuppressive that they essentially wipe out the immune system, including memory cells. In such cases, previously received vaccines may no longer work, and revaccination is recommended.

Should pregnant women receive vaccines?

The only vaccines contraindicated (not recommended) for use in pregnant women are live attenuated vaccines. This is due to the theoretical risk that live attenuated vaccines could transmit the weakened vaccine virus to the developing fetus. However, there have been no reports of any fetal infection or malformation in instances in which a live virus vaccine has been inadvertently given to a pregnant woman (i.e., in cases in which vaccines were administered before women were aware of their pregnancies).

All other types of vaccines can be safely given to pregnant women, and there is no evidence that they present any risk to the fetus. The effects of vaccines on women have been well researched, and outcomes such as spontaneous abortion, impaired fetal growth, premature birth, and congenital malformations occur no more frequently after vaccination than in the general population. In fact, vaccination has been shown to have a protective effect, decreasing the risk of some of these outcomes, including prematurity.

Currently, an inactivated virus vaccine (influenza) and a bacterial protein vaccine (Tdap) are routinely recommended for pregnant women, and new vaccines for pregnant women are under development that would be recommended exclusively for administration during pregnancy.

Do live attenuated (weakened virus or bacteria) vaccines ever cause problems in healthy individuals?

In general, live attenuated vaccines work well in healthy individuals without causing any problems. Inactivated whole virus vaccines also work well in healthy individuals. However, there is one historical exception to this rule, the "Cutter incident," which stands as both one of the largest disasters in US pharmaceutical history and a turning point for federal regulation of safe vaccines.

After Jonas Salk's polio vaccine was introduced in 1955, Cutter Laboratories in Berkeley, California, was one of multiple pharmaceutical companies licensed to manufacture this inactivated whole virus vaccine. At that time, there was no consistent oversight of vaccine manufacturing practices. In April of that year, reports emerged of paralytic polio among children who had received Cutter's polio vaccine. The Salk polio vaccine used monkey cells to grow the polio virus, which was then inactivated. An investigation after emergence of these vaccine-associated polio cases found inadequate inactivation and safety testing at Cutter, resulting in 7 of 17 batches of vaccines being contaminated with live polio virus. Production was halted, but not before thousands of doses had already been distributed. The result was an estimated 164 cases of severe paralysis and 10 deaths.

This incident transformed vaccine safety regulation and led to the establishment of a larger and more powerful Division of Biologic Standards (today's Bureau of Biologics under the FDA). Prior to the Cutter incident, very few resources were dedicated to regulating and monitoring vaccine manufacturing; today, as described in previous chapters, vaccine manufacturing procedures are tightly regulated with multiple levels of review throughout production. There have been no similar incidents since Cutter.

What happens when a vaccine-associated adverse event occurs?

As described previously, in the United States, any event that occurs after receipt of a vaccine can be reported to the VAERS surveillance system. An event may be reported by a physician or other health care provider after treating a patient with a potential vaccine-associated event. Parents or individuals may report on their own as well. The most common adverse events resolve on their own. For more significant adverse events that require ongoing care, an individual or health care provider may file a claim to the National Vaccine Injury Compensation Program (NVICP).

What is the National Vaccine Injury Compensation Program?

NVICP was established in 1986 to provide a mechanism through which individuals who experienced an adverse event related to a vaccine can be compensated. It was set up to serve as an alternative to the traditional civil courts system, in which an individual could pursue a claim directly against a vaccine manufacturer or a health care provider. NVICP is a no-fault system, meaning that compensation does not come with an admission of negligence by a vaccine manufacturer or health care provider who administered the vaccine. Compensation is instead based on a claimant's demonstration of serious injury related to a vaccine, and settlements are awarded using funds raised through an excise tax placed on all vaccines included in the program. Award amounts are designed to cover medical and other supportive care needs, as well as loss of future productivity.

In addition to providing compensation to individuals who sustained a vaccine injury, the program had additional policy goals. The first was stabilization of the vaccine market, which at the time was prohibitively risky for most developers and manufacturers due to litigation risks. This presented a prohibitive threat to a stable and sufficient vaccine supply because legal fees paid by manufacturers would lead to increases in prices of vaccines, which would in turn diminish their availability. Second, the program offered a more expedient model for case review and compensation, allowing individuals a forum to independently raise claims at less cost. Last, the program called for a vaccine safety review by the Institute of Medicine (an independent nongovernment review board now called the National Academy of Medicine), in addition to the establishment of VAERS and requisite Vaccine Information Statements distributed to all patients (or their caregivers) at the time of vaccine administration.

Which vaccines are covered by NVICP?

The program covers all vaccines recommended by the Advisory Committee on Immunization Practices for routine administration to children. This means any vaccine on the routine childhood schedule is covered, even if the vaccine is also given to adults. Vaccines that are given only to adults, such as the zoster or shingles vaccine, are not covered at this time. Although the program covers childhood vaccines, anyone who receives a vaccine can file a claim. More than half of all claims received by the program each year are from adults.

How does NVICP work?

NVICP is administered through the US Department of Health and Human Services' Health Resources and Services Administration, in cooperation with the US Department of Justice and the US Court of Federal Claims. Any individual can file a claim on behalf of him- or herself or a child, or a claim can be filed through an attorney. This claim is called a *petition*, and to be reviewed, it must be submitted within a certain period of time after the alleged injury, based on the program's established statute of limitations. Upon filing, the petition begins a review and adjudication process.

How does one qualify for compensation within NVICP?

Three paths can lead to compensation. First, a petitioner can claim an injury that is listed in the program's *vaccine injury table*. These injuries must have occurred within a certain time period after vaccination in order to be associated with the vaccine in question. The petitioner can also file a claim for an injury that is not in the vaccine injury table, but in these cases he or she must submit evidence to prove that the vaccine caused the injury. A third option for petitioners is to submit evidence that a vaccine worsened a preexisting condition. In contrast to the civil system, in which the burden of proof is "beyond a reasonable doubt," NVICP requires only "presumption of causation."

Although a petitioner has an option to pursue proof of causation for an injury submitted within the statute of limitations, not all adverse events qualify for compensation under the program. A petitioner must show that an alleged injury (1) lasted 6 months or more after receiving the vaccine in question, (2) resulted in a hospital stay or surgery, or (3) resulted in death. In addition, if the available evidence shows that the injury was caused by something other than a vaccine, the petitioner would not be eligible for compensation.

Once a petition is filed, a medical officer from the Department of Health and Human Services (HHS) performs an initial review to determine whether the previously presented criteria are met. If they are met, the case is assigned to an attorney from the Department of Justice, who in turn presents the case on behalf of HHS. Cases are heard by special masters, who are attorneys appointed by the Court of Federal Claims to review only vaccine injury cases. The special masters also review submitted evidence from the petitioner and then make a decision about compensation.

What is the NVICP vaccine injury table and what is in it?

The vaccine injury table is NVICP's list of specific injuries for which there is reliable evidence that the condition can occur after vaccination. Specific conditions are listed for each covered vaccine, along with a time frame within which the symptoms must develop to be considered a potential vaccine-related injury. However, not all covered vaccines are listed in the table; this is because there have been no injuries for a particular covered vaccine identified through safety surveillance activities. Examples of conditions currently in the table include anaphylaxis and vaccine-strain measles infection, which can manifest post-vaccination in a person with an immunodeficiency (see https://www.hrsa.gov/vaccinecompensation/vaccineinjury-table.pdf).

Because the table is informed by safety surveillance data and formal review of vaccine safety studies by the National Academy of Medicine (NAM), it can be updated over time. The latest updates were submitted in 2015 after publication of a NAM report on vaccine safety. Recommended additions included SIRVA related to any injectable vaccines, syncope, and vaccine-type varicella (chicken pox) infection in immunocompromised individuals. Adverse events such as febrile seizures are not included because they self-resolve and do not have any long-lasting effects. A review of current data can also result in removal of conditions from the table. Any individual can petition for the addition of a condition to the table and provide his or her own evidence in support of his or her request. Such petitions are reviewed by NVICP medical officers, who examine all available data related to the request, with input from subject matter experts.

Who is responsible for updating the NVICP injury table?

All proposed table additions or subtractions to the injury table must be reviewed by the Advisory Commission on Childhood Vaccines (ACCV), which was established alongside NVICP to advise the Secretary of Health and Human Services on program matters. For table updates, ACCV members review the proposed changes along with supporting data and can agree and accept the changes, disagree and recommend against the changes, or defer a recommendation until there is more time for review. The ACCV bases its decision-making on two principles: (1) The vaccine injury table should be both medically and scientifically credible (i.e., based on evidence); and (2) if there is credible evidence that both supports and rejects the proposed change (i.e., available data are equivocal or inconclusive), then any recommendation should benefit petitioners.

Occasionally, a condition can be added to the injury table for policy reasons even when the available scientific evidence does not support a causal association between a vaccine and the alleged condition. The most recent example is the decision to add GBS for influenza vaccines. With the exception of the association found with the 1976 influenza A vaccine, studies have not shown an increased risk of GBS after receipt of seasonal influenza vaccines. However, as described previously, this is a rare condition, which makes it difficult to examine in vaccine safety surveillance studies. Because influenza vaccines are different each year, there is a theoretical concern that the risk could potentially change, but this may be difficult to initially detect for an event that occurs so rarely. The proposal to add GBS to the table came with the recognition that cases not associated with vaccination may be compensated. However, it was also believed that it would be the best way to ensure that any vaccine-related cases, if they do occur, can be compensated.

Who serves on the ACCV?

The ACCV is made up of nine members: three health professionals with expertise in the health care of children, the epidemiology of childhood diseases, and vaccine adverse events; two pediatricians; three members from the general public, of whom two must represent children who have experienced a vaccine-related injury; and three attorneys, at least one of whom must have experience representing petitioners and another must represent vaccine manufacturers. All members are appointed by the Secretary of Health and Human Services and serve a minimum of 3 years. The ACCV also includes several ex officio members representing the National Institutes of Health, the CDC, and the FDA.

ACCV meetings occur quarterly, and all meetings are open to attendance and comment by the public. In addition to reviewing proposed changes to the vaccine injury table, the ACCV has recently convened working groups to revisit different aspects of the program and submitted recommendations to make the program more efficient for petitioners and more responsive to changing trends in immunization recommendations, including immunizations for expectant mothers.

How many individuals have received compensation from NVICP?

Between 2006 and 2014, a total of 3,451 petitions were reviewed by NVICP, and approximately two-thirds (2,199) were compensated. The total amount awarded was approximately $3.1

billion, with an additional $139 million paid out for attorney fees. The amount of individual awards varies based on the disability and future productivity loss associated with the alleged injury. The 3,451 petitions represent 0.000001% of the 2.5 billion doses of covered vaccines distributed during that same time period. The majority of reviewed cases are for alleged injuries after influenza vaccination among adults, showing a shift in the program over time. Influenza vaccines are recommended for all individuals older than age 6 months in the United States each year. As such, more influenza vaccine doses are administered compared to any other vaccine, and a significant proportion of these doses are administered to adults.

Compensation can be awarded via three different types of ruling: The court can concede, issue a legal decision, or settle. Concessions occur when HHS reviews all available evidence and determines that the vaccine more likely than not caused the alleged injury or that the evidence supports a table injury. (Note that in this regard, the standard for compensation applied to NVICP petitions is not the same as the standard applied in the civil court system.) One of the special masters or the US Court of Federal Claims also reviews the available evidence to issues final decisions; however, these decisions can be appealed.

Settlement, by far the most common outcome (approximately 80% of compensable claims), occurs when a petition is resolved through negotiation. This does not reflect a decision by HHS or the court that the alleged injury was caused by a vaccine. Instead, settlement is pursued if both parties would like to resolve a case quickly to minimize the expense and resource use of litigation. A settlement is not an admission by HHS or the US Court of Federal Claims that a vaccine caused an alleged injury.

When cases are not compensated or dismissed, this means that the Court reviewed the evidence and determined that the petitioner did not show that the alleged injury was caused by a vaccine or that the requirements for a table injury were not met. Cases can also be dismissed if they do not fulfill the other criteria required for submission (i.e., must be a covered vaccine). A petitioner may also choose to withdraw a claim.

Whatever the outcome, the average timeline for adjudication is 2 or 3 years.

Has NVICP compensated any autism claims?

Autism as a vaccine-associated injury has been evaluated in multiple well-designed scientific studies, all of which have shown no association between any vaccine and the risk of developing autism. The concern about vaccines as a cause of autism first arose after the 1998 publication of an article titled "Ileal-Lymphoid-Nodular Hyperplasia, Non-specific Colitis, and Pervasive Developmental Disorder in Children," whose lead author was Andrew Wakefield. The article described a series of 12 children who presented with developmental regression, or loss of developmental milestones, in the setting of gastrointestinal abnormalities. Parents of 8 of the 12 children reported that symptoms developed after receiving the MMR vaccine. Based on this small case series, Wakefield et al. alleged that MMR vaccine could result in bowel inflammation that then allows brain-damaging proteins to circulate. This hypothesis has never been demonstrated in any subsequent studies, and the article was eventually retracted by the publishing journal. Wakefield lost his medical license due to the fraudulent claims put forth in his article. Since that time, multiple rigorous studies comparing vaccinated to unvaccinated children have not shown an increased risk for autism after vaccination.

The alleged tie between vaccines and autism has nonetheless remained a concern for some parents, and in 2001 NVICP began to receive claims for autism spectrum disorder associated with MMR vaccine and/or vaccines containing thimerosal. In 2002, to most efficiently accommodate all the claims, the chief special master created an *Omnibus Autism*

Proceeding—similar to a class-action lawsuit—to adjudicate all the claims. To process all of the 5,600 petitions, the US Court of Federal Claims (which administers NVICP) established "test cases" for each of the three theories of autism causation that were represented in the claims: (1) that MMR and thimerosal together cause autism,(2) that thimerosal alone causes autism, and (3) that MMR alone causes autism. The evidence considered by the special masters was exhaustive, spanning medical studies, testimonies, and expert reports; in all three test cases, the causal link between autism and vaccines was rejected.

The omnibus cases have all been adjudicated, but some families that were part of the omnibus petition have chosen to pursue legal claims through the civil tort system.

How is information about vaccine safety from NVICP communicated?

One of the primary mechanisms for communication about potential risks associated with vaccines, as well as NVICP in general, is Vaccine Information Statements (VISs). VISs are mandated by the National Vaccine Childhood Injury Act and must be given prior to the receipt of any vaccine, including each dose of any multidose vaccine series. VISs summarize the benefits and potential risks associated with each covered vaccine and also include information about the VICP. Content is developed by the CDC and includes input from medical experts to ensure accuracy and feedback from people in the general public to ensure readability. All VISs are then reviewed and approved by the ACCV before publication. Distribution of the most up-to-date VISs is required of all vaccine providers, public or private, and must be documented in the patient's medical record. Currently, there are multiple mechanisms besides distribution of a paper copy: Providers can use a permanent, laminated office copy or present VISs on a computer monitor or other video display. VISs can be downloaded onto smartphones to be read at any time and have been translated into more than 40 languages. It is important to note that VISs are only required for vaccines covered by NVICP.

If NVICP depends on published evidence to develop the vaccine injury table and adjudicate cases, how does one evaluate the reliability and validity of a study?

Not all studies are created equal. When evaluating the risk of an outcome after an exposure such as a vaccine, one needs to be able to compare the likelihood of an event among exposed individuals to the likelihood of an event if not exposed (and ideally each group would be similar in size and characteristics). There are myriad methodological flaws that can render results from even the most well-intentioned study misleading, which is why it is important that scientists (along with governmental scientific groups such as VICP) police studies for reliability. The alternative—a poorly designed study that produces misleading or incomplete conclusions—can have a devastating effect on public understanding and acceptance of vaccines. Wakefield et al.'s retracted article is an example of this. They described a small series of cases with no comparison group and made hypotheses that were not evaluated. Still, the article's message has become wildly misrepresented in public discourse and in social media.

Who evaluates the reliability of vaccine safety studies?

There have been some recent efforts to evaluate available vaccine safety data. Published vaccine safety studies are all subject to peer review, in which scientific papers are reviewed by other scientists prior to publication to ensure their quality and validity. Sometimes individual studies on a single topic will be evaluated together to search for consistency across published results. This valuable and exhaustive research is called a comprehensive systematic review, and it is an example of the sort of work performed by the National Academy of Medicine (formerly the Institute of Medicine).

What is the National Academy of Medicine?

The National Academy of Medicine (NAM) was established by the National Academy of Sciences in 1970, initially as the Institute of Medicine, to bring together experienced scientists from a wide range of disciplines to examine topics related to public health policy, medical care, and education. It is a private, nonprofit institution, and it receives no federal funds for its work. One of NAM's primary activities is to review available research related to specific topics and to use its findings to generate recommendations and standardize practice. Requests for study topics can come from federal agencies or independent organizations, and vaccine safety has been an area of extensive NAM research during the past several years. As part of the Vaccine Injury Act, NAM was charged with reviewing literature related to vaccine adverse events, which it has done more than 10 times since 1986. One of the most recent comprehensive reports was published in 2012 and examined evidence for adverse events surrounding eight different vaccines. This work, which reviewed 12,000 published articles and was summarized in a 900-page book, led to the following recommendations for changes to the VICP vaccine injury table:

- Addition of anaphylaxis as a potential adverse event associated with MMR, meningococcal, hepatitis B, varicella, tetanus toxoid, and influenza vaccines
- Addition of both syncope and SIRVA or deltoid bursitis as potential adverse events with any injectable vaccine

Perhaps most notably, the NAM committee rejected, "with high confidence," any association between MMR vaccines and autism. Their findings also favored rejection of any association between influenza vaccines and either Bell's palsy or asthma and between MMR or pertussis-containing vaccines and type 1 diabetes.

Since this 2012 report, NAM conducted a second review evaluating the safety of the recommended childhood immunization schedule. This was requested on behalf of HHS in response to the growing frequency of requests for delayed immunization schedules, largely related to safety concerns about the number of vaccines currently recommended for any one visit. Their review of available literature focusing on adverse events related to the entire childhood schedule showed no safety concerns. There is no evidence that receiving all recommended vaccines on time is associated with autoimmune diseases, asthma, hypersensitivity or allergies, seizures, developmental disorders, or attention deficit disorder.

6

THE VACCINE SCHEDULE

The centerpiece of any immunization program is its immunization schedule, a national standard of practice for which vaccines are administered and when. The governmental groups that create immunization schedules consider a range of factors in doing so, including the vaccine's potential to improve the country's overall health and the financial implications of distributing the vaccine across the population.

Accordingly, it is no surprise that immunization schedules and programs vary by country. But who makes the decisions for individual countries, what informs their decisions, and how are recommendations communicated? These topics are the focus of this chapter. It describes the different groups that participate in the formulation and dissemination of immunization schedules and provides information to address common questions about the schedules, including the number and timing of injections and the safety of delaying vaccination. (For schedules and overviews of common child, adolescent, and adult vaccines, see the Appendix.)

Who makes the immunization schedule?

In most countries, immunization schedules are determined by a part of the public health infrastructure—typically a group of experts from medicine, public health, and vaccine research.

In the United States, this work is performed by the Advisory Committee on Immunization Practices (ACIP).

What is ACIP?

ACIP is a federal advisory committee housed within the Centers for Disease Control and Prevention (CDC) that reports to the Secretary of Health and Human Services. The committee makes recommendations to the CDC director on the immunization schedule for children, adolescents, and adults. ACIP is responsible for both the addition of new vaccines and changes to the administration of vaccines that are already on the schedule. Since 1995, the harmonized child/adolescent immunization schedule has been officially reviewed and approved by ACIP in 1995 and is now (along with the adult immunization schedule) reviewed and updated by ACIP each year. (The harmonized schedules are also reviewed by several professional societies, such as the American Academy of Pediatrics, the American Academy of Family Practitioners, the American College of Physicians, and the American College of Obstetricians and Gynecologists; as a matter of practice, the harmonized schedules are not published until all of these groups have given their approval.)

Another important function of ACIP is determining which vaccines will be included in the Vaccines for Children (VFC) program, which, as detailed in Chapter 4, was established in 1993 to provide free vaccines for any child younger than age 18 years who is uninsured, eligible for Medicaid, of American Indian or Alaska Native descent, or underinsured and receiving care at a federally qualified health center. To ensure that vaccines included in the recommended schedule are accessible to all children, the vaccines recommended by ACIP for routine use are also included in the VFC program.

When was ACIP first established?

Early in the development of the immunization program in the United States, the public health service would bring together groups of experts as needed to make decisions about which vaccines to give routinely and when. However, as the immunization program expanded with more new vaccines, it was clear that an established group of advisors outside of the federal government was needed to provide continuity and rigor in decision-making. This led to a proposal to create ACIP in 1964 through the Public Health Service Act. This legislation authorized the US Department of Health and Human Services to provide assistance to states to prevent and control communicable diseases. The Act also authorized establishment of advisory committees. At that time, the Committee's charge was to advise the Surgeon General on the most effective public health use of "preventive agents" to control communicable diseases. The Committee was asked to focus on immunization schedules, dosage and administration route of vaccines, contraindications for use, and decisions about which groups of individuals should receive a vaccine.

Initially, ACIP consisted of eight members appointed by the Secretary of Health from pediatrics, epidemiology, immunology, and public health. There were also three liaison organizations (the American Academy of Pediatrics Committee on Infectious Diseases, the American Medical Association, and the Advisory Committee on Immunization from Canada) and ex officio members from other federal government entities involved in vaccine development, including the US Food and Drug Administration and the National Institutes of Health.

In 1972, ACIP underwent a major change when it became a federal advisory committee. As per the Federal Advisory Committee Act, this led to open meetings, increased public involvement, and reporting requirements. At this time, the Committee changed from reporting to the Surgeon General to reporting to the Secretary of Health through the CDC. The number of members also increased to include experts in the social sciences, law and ethics, as well as one consumer—a member of the public who represents patients and families who receive or are considering immunization. ACIP currently has 15 voting members, all of whom are employed outside of the federal government, and it liaises with 29 related organizations and 8 ex officio members in forming its recommendations.

How are ACIP members selected?

ACIP members are selected for a 4-year term, and candidates must be nominated. Recommendations for new members may come from professional organizations, former or current ACIP members, or the general public. Open positions are announced widely to encourage a transparent and inclusive process, and candidates follow a standard application process similar to any job application process. Candidates cannot be employees of the Department of Health and Human Services.

The ACIP Steering Committee reviews all applications and then selects and forwards two nominees for each open position to the director of the CDC for review. The director performs an additional review of each nominee and forwards applications to the Secretary of Health and Human Services, who makes the final decision. Before they are advanced to this stage, applications are closely reviewed for any potential conflicts of interest, including financial relationships or lobbying relationships with any commercial entities involved in vaccine development or manufacturing. For example, if a nominee has any relationship or interest in a specific vaccine, that person would not be considered for appointment to ACIP. This would include anyone who holds a patent for a vaccine or is employed by or has an immediate family member employed by a vaccine manufacturer. Even among sitting members, conflicts of interest continue to be monitored closely: All members must submit a financial report each year for review by the Office of Government Ethics and publicly announce all work related to vaccines at every regular and working group meeting. If concern for potential conflicts of interest among members exists, the relevant member may not be permitted to participate in certain aspects of the committee's work. If a major conflict arises, a member will be asked to resign.

What criteria are used to select members for ACIP?

ACIP membership decisions take into account qualifications and experience in an individual's given field. Medical and public health professionals must have an advanced professional degree, such as an M.D. or R.N., along with board certification in their specialty. They must also demonstrate a commitment to participate in all regularly scheduled and emergency meetings and show comfort contributing to discussions in front of a large public audience. ACIP meetings occur three times annually in Atlanta, Georgia; are typically attended by 300–400 people (including members of the public); and are broadcast on the Internet. Efforts are made to ensure that ACIP members are diverse in terms of geographic home, professional background, gender, race, and ethnicity. The 15-member voting committee includes a "lay member"—an individual from the general public to represent the perspectives of families and parents. The overall goal is to have proceedings represent a range of perspectives to inform recommendations.

Are members of ACIP paid?

Voting ACIP members are considered Special Government Employees and have the option of receiving a $250 honorarium for each meeting day. Nonvoting members do not receive compensation for their time participating in meetings, but they do receive reimbursement for travel expenses to attend in-person meetings. Voting members also receive travel reimbursement.

How does ACIP make decisions about the immunization schedule?

ACIP members generally possess a thorough and up-to-date grounding in epidemiology and vaccine research and science, and their knowledge is supplemented with data and research from the CDC and working groups convened to inform the committee. In addition to considering factors such as epidemiology, vaccine safety, and results from clinical trials, ACIP members also review economic analyses about vaccine costs and costs associated with adding a vaccine to the immunization program. Although these cost considerations are not new, ACIP's charter was updated in 2004 to require formal reference to any economic analyses when presenting data in support of its recommendations. The committee's use of economic data was standardized through the 2008 publication titled "Guidance for Health Economics Studies Presented to the ACIP," and today cost considerations are considered as important as any factor in proposing changes to the vaccine schedule.

ACIP also receives information from a range of stakeholders with experience with particular vaccine-preventable diseases or the vaccines themselves. Representatives from the World Health Organization or other national immunization organizations are regularly invited to share perspectives or expertise. In addition, all ACIP meetings are open to the public, and individuals are invited to give public comment. This gives ACIP members exposure to the range of values and perspectives related to a particular vaccine that may have implications for the acceptability of their recommendations.

ACIP considers the previously mentioned perspectives to recommend (1) whether a vaccine should be given routinely to everyone within a certain age group or only under special circumstances (i.e., individuals with certain risk factors), (2) how and when the vaccine should be given (i.e., at what ages and intervals), and (3) who should not receive the vaccine. Instructions for age groups, dosing, and intervals between doses generally follow the indications that were approved for licensure, but ACIP sometimes makes additional recommendations that were not included with the approved indications. For example, the tetanus, diphtheria, acellular pertussis (Tdap) vaccine is recommended by ACIP for all pregnant women during each pregnancy to prevent pertussis in infants. However, because Tdap during pregnancy was not a part of the initial clinical trials for the vaccine's licensure, this was an "off-label" recommendation. To inform their decision, ACIP reviewed available evidence from other studies that supported the safety and effectiveness of Tdap administration during pregnancy.

What kind of evidence does ACIP use?

As mentioned previously, ACIP now applies a systematic approach to ensure that it is using the best available evidence. Since 2010, this approach has been guided by a few key principles, including transparency and the consideration of both community and individual health perspectives when evaluating the potential impact of vaccination. Transparency is achieved by including multiple stakeholders as active participants in meetings as well as public engagement. Community considerations might include herd immunity, in which a certain level of vaccination in a community can prevent transmission. Evidence is evaluated using an approach that measures the quality of evidence by evaluating the type of available studies, their validity, and the consistency of results.

How long does it take for ACIP to develop recommendations?

Because ACIP reviews such an exhaustive amount of information, the development of a new recommendation can take several months, even years. After an initial review, ACIP may request additional data that can take time to compile. Ensuring that there is adequate opportunity for stakeholders to provide input can also take time. Because strength of evidence is important, significant attention is paid to compiling reliable information to guide decision-making.

What happens after a recommendation is made?

Once ACIP votes to implement a recommendation, it is then officially reviewed and approved by the director of the CDC, who in turn communicates the recommendation to the Secretary and Assistant Secretary of Health and Human Services. The recommendation is then published in the CDC's official periodical, *Morbidity and Mortality Weekly Report*, which is widely read and represents the recommendation's official dissemination. However, word generally begins to spread before that time. Any recommendations passed by ACIP are generally summarized in a press release at the end of each meeting, and these get picked up in popular media. Professional organizations may also communicate new recommendations to their members.

How are ACIP recommendations actually implemented?

After immunization recommendations come from ACIP (via the CDC), implementation takes place through state and local health departments and individual health care providers. The immunization schedule communicates to clinics which vaccines to order; in the case of publicly funded immunization programs, state or local health departments do the ordering. Thus, communication of the schedule is important, and in turn health departments, clinics, and individual care providers (including physicians) are depended on to apply it.

Do states have their own vaccine advisory committees?

Some states have formed their own advisory committees to help guide implementation of federal recommendations in their state. These groups may help tailor decisions surrounding immunization requirements for school entry or financing for individuals who are not covered under federal programs such as the VFC. In other words, state vaccine committees adapt routine schedules to their own state's needs and resources.

Why is there only one recommended schedule?

Multiple recommendations for an immunization schedule existed in the United States until 1995. Before 1995, professional organizations such as the American Academy of Pediatrics (AAP) published their own schedules, largely based on ACIP recommendations but with occasional deviations. (For example, when a second booster dose of the measles, mumps, and rubella vaccine was first recommended in the early 1990s, ACIP recommended administration at age 4–6 years to coincide with the administration of other booster doses; the AAP recommended the booster for 11- and 12-year-olds because most outbreaks at that time were taking place in middle school- and high school-aged children.) The different schedules posed a challenge to pediatricians, who had to choose sides in their messaging and recommendations to patients. In 1994 ACIP, AAP, and the American Academy of Family Physicians (AAFP) resolved to publish one harmonized, easy-to-understand schedule for routinely recommended childhood vaccines, balancing both programmatic concerns and epidemiology. ACIP similarly liaises with the American College of Physicians, the AAFP, and the American College of Obstetricians and Gynecologists to publish a harmonized schedule for adult immunizations.

What is wrong with following a different schedule, such as spreading out vaccines, rather than following the recommended vaccine schedule?

Spreading out vaccines means that some vaccine doses will be delayed. The primary concern with regard to delaying vaccines is that it increases the amount of time during which a child is unprotected and can contract a host of serious diseases that could threaten his or her life or, at minimum, make the child very sick. In addition, a more spread-out vaccine schedule fails to make use of an expansive body of scientific research that has distilled the vaccine schedule into one that both maximizes immunity when risk is highest and guarantees that the vaccines work well together. In choosing a schedule that has not been evaluated in the same way, there is no guarantee that the vaccines will work most effectively.

Some parents may request a delayed schedule because of concerns that receiving several vaccines at the same time may overwhelm the immune system or be too stressful or painful for their child. However, spreading out vaccines may not necessarily produce less stress, especially if they are given in a way that results in fewer doses given more frequently: Studies have demonstrated that infants who receive only one vaccine produce as much cortisol, a stress hormone, as infants who receive two vaccines at the same time.

Do the number and combinations of vaccines given in the recommended schedule overwhelm the immune system?

In short, no. Some parents express concern that the immunization schedule is too crowded and may be too much for a child's immune system. Vaccines work by presenting antigens to the body that stimulate an immune response. It is important to remember that these antigens are a small part of the bacteria or virus the vaccine protects against. The number of antigens included in vaccines, even if a child receives four or five vaccines at one time, is much smaller than the number of antigens in the body during an actual infection—or even from the many allergens and bacteria in the environment encountered on a daily basis.

How do we know the recommended schedule is safe?

From overwhelming the immune system to potentially contributing to the development of neurodevelopmental or autoimmune disorders, many people have questions about the impact of giving several vaccines that will all stimulate the immune system together.

Vaccine safety is one of the many pieces of information ACIP considers when it is developing recommendations. Part of the cost of vaccination that is considered against the benefits of it is any potential side effect associated with vaccination.

Because side effects are monitored closely in all of the studies required for a vaccine to be licensed, this information is available to ACIP. These safety studies include an evaluation of any potential side effects when vaccines are given together.

Concerns about the development of neurodevelopmental or autoimmune disorders have also been rigorously addressed by several studies that have evaluated the risk for some of these outcomes after completing the recommended vaccine series. As summarized in Chapter 5, the National Academy of Medicine authored what is regarded as the most authoritative evaluation of evidence—a systematic review of all available literature on this topic. Its conclusions endorsed "with high confidence" the safety of the recommended immunization schedule.

How do immunization programs keep track of who needs what?

Once recommendations have been communicated, providers cannot implement them without knowing who is due for a vaccine and when. All immunization programs have some standard of documenting when a vaccine was delivered and to whom. In the United States, immunization history is a part of all medical records, and immunizations are often reported to a registry maintained by a state or local health department that keeps track of all the vaccines delivered to individuals who reside within a certain area. All states and even some large cities have an immunization registry. Although the completeness of all registry data can vary, its consolidation serves to both identify individuals who are due for vaccines and measure immunization rates to identify gaps across a population.

7

LAWS AND STANDARD PRACTICES FOR VACCINE ADMINISTRATION

Despite the fact that vaccines have been shown to drastically improve health outcomes at both individual and public health levels, their implementation as a civic requirement has been a longtime source of conflict. At the heart of this issue is the dual nature of vaccines as both a personal choice and a matter of public interest: They work not only by preventing infection in vaccinated individuals but also by preventing transmission to other people. Vaccination is an individual decision that affects others, which puts vaccine policy squarely in the hotly contested domain of public health policy. Public health policy affects our lives (and, some would argue, betters our lives) in many ways. For example, no-smoking laws in restaurants prevent exposure to second-hand smoke, just as requisite Board of Health licensure reduces the risk of food-borne illnesses. In each of these cases, an individual liberty is curtailed for public good—to prevent disease within a community. Vaccine policy is an example of the tension that can exist between public good and individual liberty.

What is vaccine policy?

The term *vaccine policy* refers to a wide range of issues, including public vaccine requirements, licensure requirements to ensure safety, recommendations for the use of vaccines, financing strategies for programs such as Vaccines for Children that increase access to immunizations, and outreach programs to increase awareness about vaccines. The goal of vaccine policy is to achieve a sufficiently high immunization rate within a community, thereby reducing disease risk by preventing transmission—that is, achieving *herd immunity*. The crux of many countries' vaccine policies is immunization requirements. This could manifest as requirements for individuals within a community to be vaccinated during a disease outbreak or as a condition of participation in certain activities in which the risk of exposure to a vaccine-preventable disease is high. For example, in the United States, all 50 states require that students receive certain vaccines before entering kindergarten or middle school. In many hospitals, health care workers are required to receive certain vaccines as a condition of their employment.

What are the historical and legal precedents for mandatory vaccination?

Conflict regarding vaccine requirements has been present in the United States since the end of the 18th century, when mandatory vaccination against smallpox was first imposed by cities facing outbreaks. This particular issue would eventually result in the 1905 Supreme Court case *Jacobsen v. Massachusetts*, in which Jacobsen refused to comply with a State of Massachusetts requirement to receive smallpox vaccine or incur a $5 fine, citing intrusion on individual liberty. The court upheld the constitutionality of vaccine mandates based on the premise that a state can compel immunization "to protect itself against an epidemic of disease which threatens the safety of its members":

> The liberty secured by the Constitution of the United States . . . does not import an absolute right . . . to be wholly freed from restraint. There are manifold restraints

to which every person is necessarily subject for the common good. . . . Society based on the rule that each one is a law unto himself would soon be confronted with anarchy and disorder.

In *Zucht v. King* (1922), the Supreme Court unanimously upheld a local government mandate requiring vaccination for public school attendance. This gave precedent for state and local municipalities to develop their own standards for immunization requirements, allowable exemptions, and enforcement mechanisms. Later, in *Prince v. Massachusetts* (1944), the Court's ruling had sweeping implications for parents' right to refuse vaccination for their children based on religious beliefs. The case centered on a Jehovah's Witness parent who claimed the right to have her 9-year-old child distribute religious pamphlets on the street—work that the Court ruled was a violation of child labor laws. The Court ruled that religious freedom did not trump child labor laws, and in doing so also commented on vaccine refusal and religious beliefs:

> [A parent] cannot claim freedom from compulsory vaccination for the child any more than for himself on religious grounds. The right to practice religion freely does not include the liberty to expose the community to infectious disease. Parents may be free to become martyrs themselves; but it does not follow they are free . . . to make martyrs of their children.

This latter case also speaks to equal protection and the rights of the child: According to the 14th Amendment's Equal Protection Clause, every person, including a child, should have equal protection from harm. Because vaccines are meant to prevent harm from vaccine-preventable diseases, the clause implies that a decision not to vaccinate could violate a child's right to be protected. In fact, in two of the states that do not allow

nonmedical exemptions from school immunization requirements, their respective state Supreme Courts ruled that such
exemptions violate the 14th Amendment.

Even with these precedents, immunization requirements
for school entry did not become a central feature of US vaccine
policy until the 1960s and 1970s, when states began to enact
legislation in response to measles outbreaks among schoolchildren. Prior to that time, many health departments would
only require immunization as an emergency action to stop outbreaks; here, state legislatures required vaccination as a condition of school attendance to *prevent* outbreaks.

What are the basic arguments that support immunization requirements?

The elimination of many major childhood diseases from
schools and communities is one good argument for requiring
vaccines: Vaccine requirements generally lead to high immunization rates. More people are protected, so less disease exists,
and vaccine-preventable diseases have less opportunity to
spread. Because vaccines have demonstrated their effectiveness at preventing disease for an individual, and because the
decision to vaccinate (or not vaccinate) has the potential to
affect other people, immunization requirements uphold the
ethical principles of *beneficence* (providing good) and *nonmaleficence* (do no harm) while also promoting *equity* (personal
justice through a collective endeavor).

What are the basic arguments against immunization requirements?

The argument that vaccines promote equity is countered
by an argument that vaccination's benefits can be achieved
without individual participation: If an individual in a highly
immunized community chooses to not receive a vaccine, he
or she will still be insulated from the disease by virtue of the

community's collective immunization. Some may also argue that vaccination does not uphold nonmaleficence principles if there are concerns about vaccine safety.

On a more practical level, public pushback against vaccine requirements has increased as the threat of vaccine-preventable diseases appears less imminent. In this way, contemporary opinions regarding vaccines have suffered because vaccines have been effective in reducing the visibility of disease. This has partly accounted for the growth of vaccine resistance (discussed in Chapter 8), as concerns about vaccine safety have eclipsed concerns about disease. To this point, it is important to remember that vaccines must meet a very high bar for safety in order to be licensed and recommended—and must fulfill the principle of nonmaleficence to justify a requirement.

There are also ethical principles that immunization requirements violate, the principle of autonomy. An individual ultimately has the right to choose whether he or she wants to be vaccinated, and even the existence of vaccine requirements can be met by an individual decision to not vaccinate and accept whatever consequence may be imposed. For school-entry requirements, this may mean that a child cannot enroll in school; for workplace requirements, an individual may lose his or her employment. In this way, the choice is not entirely free, which violates the principle of autonomy. One can also argue that vaccines are coercive because the cost of the choice may be so high that it does not really seem like a choice.

What kinds of vaccine requirements are employed in the United States?

The cornerstone of US vaccine policy is the school-entry requirement, which mandates that all students without a medical contraindication receive certain vaccines prior to entering kindergarten (or, in some states, middle school). The requirements for specific vaccines vary by state, and they apply only to schools that receive state or local funding—although most private and parochial schools have their own vaccine requirements as well. (An exception to this public–private divide is California, which relatively recently passed a school-entry vaccination requirement that applies to public and private schools and mandates that unvaccinated children without an acceptable exemption must be homeschooled.)

For schools that require vaccines, parents must provide immunization records documenting receipt of required vaccines by a certain date at the beginning of the school year or submit an exemption. Without an exemption, an unvaccinated child would not be permitted to remain in school. However, the enforcement of requirements varies by school; immunization records must be reported to the state by a certain date, but what happens to underimmunized children who do not have an exemption is ultimately at the discretion of the school. A school-entry requirement is not the same as fully compulsory vaccination: It is a condition of attendance at a publicly funded school, but it is not an absolute requirement because there are opportunities to opt out or to choose a non-public school that may not have similar requirements.

What are the benefits of school-entry requirements?

School-entry requirements originated to minimize the incidence of vaccine-preventable diseases among school-aged children, who by virtue of their proximity to one anther are at particular risk for exposure in a school setting. Many vaccine-preventable childhood diseases are most prevalent in young children, and a school setting provides many opportunities for transmission.

School-entry requirements also reap ancillary benefits. From a public health policy perspective, requiring vaccination for school entry is an effective way to ensure high immunization rates in a community. When vaccines are required for school entry, it prompts immunization programs to ensure that required vaccines are accessible to all children, which means that school-entry requirements promote equity in immunization rates. In addition, school requirements shape how we view vaccines: Those that are required may seem more important and may receive a stronger recommendation from providers, whereas those that are not required may not be prioritized in the same way. Last, requirements make vaccination a default from which parents must opt out; disease prevention is the norm.

Interestingly, the United States is one of the few countries to require vaccination for school entry. Other countries may deliver vaccines in schools, or prevent unvaccinated students from attending schools during times of outbreak, but do not have a specific requirement for school attendance.

How does one opt out of school-entry requirements?

Although all states have school-entry requirements, every state also allows some form of exemption in recognition of individual freedom of choice and to support vaccine safety. There are three exemption types: medical, religious, and philosophical. Their application differs significantly across states.

All 50 states allow a medical exemption for children who have a medical contraindication to a required vaccine—for example, a compromised immune system that would prevent a child from receiving live virus vaccines such as measles, mumps, and rubella (MMR). Any such medical condition would require documentation and verification from a health care provider. In three states (Mississippi, West Virginia, and California), medical exemptions are the only type of vaccine exemption permitted.

Religious and philosophical exemptions are less standard across states. Currently, 47 states allow religious exemptions, and 18 states also allow philosophical exemptions (Figure 7.1). Both religious and philosophical exemptions are defined broadly and can encompass any belief, moral or religious, that goes against vaccination.

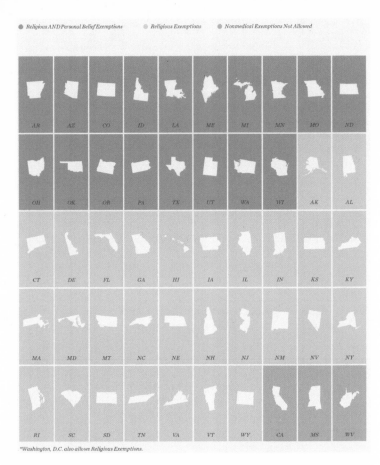

Figure 7.1 Vaccine Exemption Types by State, 2016 (extracted from http://bit.ly/
E2A_AddressingVaccineHesitancy)

Within these broad categories of exemption, a wide range
of regulations govern their invocation by parents. In some
states, a religious exemption can only be claimed if a parent
submits a written statement from a religious leader indicating that vaccination is against their doctrine. In other states,
a religious exemption can be applied to any belief, moral or
religious, that does not support vaccination, and all that is

required is a written statement from the parent indicating why he or she does not want his or her child vaccinated. Other states may require documentation of vaccine education and signed acknowledgment that the parent and child have been informed of the risks of not vaccinating.

What impact do exemption policies have on immunization rates?

As of 2015, nonmedical exemption rates varied from 0.4% to 6.2% among states that allow religious and/or philosophical exemptions. Rates can vary even more substantially across communities within states: In 2010, exemption rates among counties in Washington state ranged from 1.0% to 25.3%. Recent studies have evaluated how different exemption policies can impact both exemption rates and the risk of disease outbreaks. These studies categorized exemption policies as "easy" (i.e., requiring only parental statement), "medium" (i.e., requiring health care provider signature), or "difficult" (i.e., requiring notarization) and then examined exemption rates and disease occurrence in the respective regions. Results showed that the more difficult the exemption policy, the lower the exemption rate for that particular state. In counties and census tracts with higher exemption rates, there have been more outbreaks of vaccine-preventable diseases such as pertussis and measles. For example, children with vaccine exemptions were found to be at significantly greater risk (35 times greater) for acquiring measles compared to fully vaccinated children, and as the county vaccine-exemption rate increased, so did the incidence of measles. During a 2010 outbreak of pertussis (whooping cough) in California, census areas associated with a cluster of nonmedical vaccine exemptions were 2.5 times more likely to also have a cluster of pertussis cases. In New York state, counties with average exemption rates that exceed 1% have a significantly higher incidence of pertussis.

Have exemption laws changed over time?

The past decade has seen efforts from both sides of the vaccine-exemption issue to either tighten or loosen vaccine-exemption laws. Between 2009 and 2012, 31 bills were introduced across 18 states to make it easier to obtain exemptions. None of these bills passed, but exemption rates have increased in some states as more parents pursue requests under existing regulations. During the same time period, 5 states introduced bills to make it more difficult to achieve exemptions—three of these passed.

Exemption requirements came into the public conscious in earnest following a 2015 measles outbreak that originated at California's Disneyland and spread to several other states, eventually affecting 147 individuals, the majority of whom were unvaccinated or had unknown immunization status. Although larger outbreaks had occurred in smaller communities, a measles outbreak associated with a highly public and frequently traveled location drew attention to the potential impact of exemption policies on disease risk and spurred the introduction of legislation to curtail exemptions in some states, especially because the majority of individuals infected in the outbreak were unvaccinated due to choice or because they had medical conditions that precluded them from being vaccinated.

What has happened with vaccine-exemption legislation since the 2015 measles outbreak?

Since the 2015 measles outbreak, California has passed a highly publicized bill to remove all philosophical and religious exemptions for school-entry requirements that would apply to both public and private schools, and today children who are unvaccinated and lack a medical exemption must be homeschooled (with some exceptions for children with special needs). Rhode Island passed a law removing its philosophical exemption, and now the state only allows medical and religious exemptions in cases in which documentation can be provided. As of 2017, nine states have an educational mandate that requires that parents receive education about the risks and benefits of vaccines if they wish to pursue a nonmedical exemption.

What are other types of mandatory immunization policies?

Other settings in which immunization may be required for participation include health care facilities and daycare centers, where the risk of employees' exposure to vaccine-preventable diseases (and subsequent transmission to others, especially vulnerable individuals) is high. An example of this sort of policy is influenza vaccination requirements for health care workers. Most health care settings in the United States require that workers have documented receipt of hepatitis B and MMR vaccines at the time of employment. However, influenza vaccination, which needs to take place annually, has been a larger challenge.

Health care workers (HCWs) have been identified as a priority group for influenza vaccination for several years. The practice of HCW vaccination has been widely endorsed by multiple professional and public health societies domestically and internationally, and most health care institutions have implemented initiatives aimed at vaccinating their entire workforce against influenza. Multiple factors have been cited in support of HCW influenza vaccination, none more compelling than its potential to protect patients who may be at higher risk for severe influenza disease.

Influenza is highly contagious and easily transmitted, which means that HCWs caring for patients infected with the virus can get sick themselves and then spread it to others. In addition, an HCW is more likely to come into contact with patients who either cannot receive influenza vaccine or in whom the vaccine does not work as well, so their immunity to the virus is paramount. Influenza vaccination also protects HCWs by decreasing the likelihood that they will get sick, miss work, and potentially infect others in their households. For all of these reasons, HCW influenza vaccination is considered a patient safety strategy and also upholds some of the ethical principles discussed previously in this chapter.

Nonetheless, vaccination rates among HCWs have remained persistently low for a variety of reasons, including beliefs about vaccine effectiveness, perceived risk of developing influenza and transmitting it to others, and lack of convenient access to the vaccines. Health care institutions have employed a wide range of strategies to overcome these barriers but have continued to have difficulty significantly raising rates. This has led to the adoption of more stringent immunization requirements for HCWs, including, but not limited to, loss of employment in cases of noncompliance.

Do any other settings require immunizations?

The US Military Services employ mandatory immunization policies for their personnel. Specific requirements depend on one's deployment and subsequent exposure risk, so in addition to vaccines recommended for all adults, some military personnel may also be required to receive smallpox or anthrax vaccines. Vaccination is a condition of service for active duty personnel unless a medical exemption is confirmed.

Some college and university campuses require that students receive certain vaccines prior to enrollment, especially if students will reside in campus housing, in which the risk of exposure to vaccine-preventable diseases may be higher. The meningococcal vaccine is an example of a required vaccine at some colleges and universities. These requirements may be enforced through strategies such as a registration hold on any student lacking documentation of required vaccines.

Vaccines may also be required for certain types of travel and immigration, including individuals coming from countries where yellow fever is common (typically sub-Saharan Africa and areas of South America). Yellow fever is a mosquito-borne illness that can cause a severe, sometimes fatal, infection, and any country that is home to the type of carrier mosquito may require documentation of vaccination to prevent the import of yellow fever. Without a certificate of vaccination, travelers can be denied entry when a requirement is in place. For individuals immigrating to the United States, most of the vaccines included on the routine schedule are required for entry at the time of the immigration medical exam.

What other policy strategies are used to increase immunization rates?

Alternative public health policy approaches may be employed to increase immunization rates. These may include communication strategies such as public service announcements and other media campaigns to raise awareness about vaccines or vaccine-preventable diseases. Governments may also institute policies aimed at increasing access to vaccines as another way to increase rates—for example, by funding policies such as the Vaccines for Children program or through policies that allow for vaccine delivery in non-health care settings such as pharmacies and schools. Financial incentives to vaccinate (or penalties for not vaccinating) have also been utilized. In Australia, families receive a nontaxable cash payment for each child aged 18–24 months or 4 or 5 years who meets immunization requirements. In Slovenia, parents who do not have their children receive required vaccines must pay a fine. Other countries have offered nutrition services in tandem with vaccination as an incentive, or they may employ immunization campaigns and send health care workers to homes and other community settings to reach as many people as possible.

Are there other countries that have mandatory immunization policies?

Different countries employ a wide range of public health policy strategies to increase immunization rates, but few have mandatory immunization requirements similar to those in the United States. As mentioned previously, Slovenia requires vaccination against nine designated diseases by age 18 months or families face a fine. Three Canadian provinces require certain vaccines for school entry, but like the United States, parents may request a medical, religious, or philosophical exemption. Other countries have mandatory immunization policies for specific circumstances: Latvia requires vaccines only for immunization providers and state institutions, but it requires all health care providers to obtain signatures from patients and parents who refuse a vaccine; Belgium requires only the polio vaccine. The World Health Organization does not maintain any official policy on mandatory vaccinations but acknowledges that mandatory policies may be pursued in some settings if there are decreasing immunization rates or an outbreak is observed.

Are there ways to prevent the transmission of vaccine-preventable diseases other than vaccination?

As long as there are exemptions to vaccine requirements, there will always be individuals who are not vaccinated. Thus, other measures are sometimes taken to reduce the risk of exposure and transmission. For example, unvaccinated children may not be permitted to attend school during an outbreak or if there is a known exposure to a vaccine-preventable disease. Unvaccinated children may also be quarantined (isolated from other people) for a certain period of time to ensure that they do not develop the disease and infect others. Health care workers who are not vaccinated against influenza may not be able to work with certain patients or may be asked to wear a mask during influenza season to minimize the chances that they could infect others. These are all alternative strategies to vaccination, but they do come with restrictions in activity.

What do health care providers do if patients or families refuse a vaccine?

In recent surveys, the majority of pediatricians report at least one vaccine refusal per month, and a full 90% report requests to spread out recommended vaccines. When this happens, a pediatrician can accept the request and continue to provide care or can provide counseling and document the patient's refusal—probably with plans to revisit the discussion at another time. Some pediatricians may accept a request to spread out vaccines even if they do not agree with the decision; in other instances, practices may have a policy to dismiss families who refuse vaccines or do not follow the recommended vaccine schedule. This can be a difficult decision for pediatricians, who may believe that delaying or not administering a vaccine goes against their ethical obligation to provide the standard of care and that by caring for patients who are outside the vaccine schedule, the safety of other patients in their practice may be compromised. On the other hand, pediatricians may want to maintain the relationship they have with families to continue providing other aspects of care that are a part of health maintenance.

Are health care providers liable for vaccine refusal in any way?

A health care provider may feel personally responsible if a child in his or her practice acquires a vaccine-preventable disease from an unvaccinated child or if an unvaccinated child acquires a vaccine-preventable disease. This is why vaccine refusal is generally documented in a patient's medical record, typically with a statement confirming that the parent was counseled of the risks and benefits of vaccination and that he or she expressed an understanding of the risks of not vaccinating.

Can health care providers ask a patient or family to leave the practice if they refuse vaccines?

In general, the health care provider's goal is to maintain a relationship with a patient or family so that there is a platform for continued dialogue about vaccination and to continue to deliver health care to the child. However, if a parent's or patient's vaccine refusal or delay interferes with a provider's trust or ability to provide care in general, the provider may opt to refer the patient to another practice. This guidance is provided for in a policy statement by the American Academy of Pediatrics published in 2016. In some instances, families search for a practice with a clear immunization policy that includes dismissal. Other families may search for a provider who indicates that he or she is willing to offer different immunization schedules.

What are the potential consequences of family dismissal? Some may argue that dismissal results in a lost opportunity to provide ongoing counseling about vaccines (along with other aspects of care). In addition, if certain clinics or practices are more likely to accept families who request to delay or refuse certain vaccines, there could be clustering of unvaccinated and undervaccinated children in such practices, which could potentially increase risk of a vaccine-preventable disease outbreak.

Why would different providers have different immunization policies, especially if there is one routine recommended schedule?

There are many reasons why a health care provider may decide to accept alternative vaccine schedules. Often, the request is based on the parent's or patient's vaccine safety concerns, which the health care provider could potentially address. Continuing to work with a family presents an opportunity to provide education to address concerns while maintaining a relationship with the family or individual patient. On the other hand, some providers may believe that immunization is a central element of the care, and if they are not able to provide recommended vaccines, they are not providing standard of care and are potentially placing a child at risk of a preventable disease. This may seem like a violation of the ethical principle nonmaleficence, or "first do no harm." Some health care providers may have their own beliefs about vaccines and question vaccine safety and efficacy. Although the routine immunization schedule is the same throughout the US health care landscape, the experience, training, and vaccine education of individual providers are not. This creates an opening for different beliefs to arise, which likely drives the differences in practices across health care providers.

Are individuals who choose not to vaccinate themselves or their children ever held responsible for exposing other people to vaccine-preventable diseases?

Bioethicists and legal experts have debated the question of individual liability for the potential harm associated with a decision not to vaccinate. Consider the following scenario: Parents of a young child are concerned about the safety of the MMR vaccine and choose not to vaccinate their child. The family then visits Disneyland during the outset of the 2015 measles outbreak, and then returns home. Their child soon develops fever and cold symptoms (the first signs of measles before the rash develops), so they visit their pediatrician. In the waiting room, there are several children, some of whom are infants younger than 1 year old who are too young to receive the MMR vaccine. One of these infants develops measles, gets very sick and ends up in the hospital for several days. The parents of the affected infant believe that the parents of the unvaccinated young child are responsible for what happened. Can the affected parents take legal action?

Under civil liability law, one could make an argument for holding the parents of the unvaccinated child responsible for the other child(ren)'s illness. The test for this case would be: *has a legal duty been breached?* Some courts have held that any individual who knowingly has a highly infectious disease has a duty to take appropriate precautions, either to warn others or to prevent transmission. In the Disneyland example, however, that would mean that the parents *knew* their child was infected with a highly infectious disease, which is not clear.

The other consideration here is a parent's ability to establish causation: He or she would need to prove that the measles virus infecting the unvaccinated child was the same virus that infected the infant. If the unvaccinated child were the only measles case in the community, it would be easier to link the two cases; the older child would be the only source of the infant's exposure. The more common the infection, the more difficult it is to establish causation.

In some instances, courts have held individuals liable for knowingly transmitting an infectious disease to others (e.g.,, herpes infection). No legal precedent exists for holding an unvaccinated child liable for the exposure of another child to an infectious disease. However, in some cases, parents have been held criminally liable for harm to their own children by refusing to seek out medical care when their children developed a treatable infection (*Commonwealth of Pennsylvania v. Schaible*, 2014). In the case of *Commonwealth of Pennsylvania v. Schaible*, infection resulted in death. In some jurisdictions, a court may also pursue a charge of neglect if a parent refuses to vaccinate his or her child in the setting of an outbreak.

Rather than debating liability, some have proposed a "no-fault" approach as a means of imposing a cost on the decision not to vaccinate. In practice, this would constitute a tax or fee equal to the estimated cost of not vaccinating (i.e., the public costs associated with a vaccine-preventable disease) and would be similar to imposing higher registration fees for motorcycle riders who do not wear helmets. In these proposals, funds collected from such fees could be used to help cover costs in the event of a disease outbreak. Others have proposed increasing insurance premiums for unvaccinated individuals.

8

VACCINE HESITANCY

Questions regarding the benefits of vaccines and their safety have persisted since vaccines were first introduced during the 18th century. As widespread vaccination has caused the prevalence of vaccine-preventable diseases to decrease, public concern for the threat of these diseases has decreased, too. This has created a vacuum in which facts and non-facts mix, and some of the loudest voices have been those that question the purpose and efficacy of vaccines. This has given rise to what is known as *vaccine hesitancy*.

Vaccine hesitancy is the primary reason cited in exemption requests to school-based immunization requirements in the United States. Challenges to vaccine acceptance also affect other regions of the world, including a heralded 2003 incident in which five states in Nigeria boycotted a polio vaccination campaign (mounted in the face of ongoing polio cases in the region) due to fears that the polio vaccine was a vehicle for a sterilization program led by the West. After publication of the Wakefield et al.' article in 1998 alleging that measles, mumps, and rubella (MMR) vaccines may be linked to autism, MMR immunization rates in the United Kingdom and other European Union countries decreased significantly, resulting in measles outbreaks, particularly in France. The Ministry of Health in Japan withdrew its human papillomavirus (HPV) vaccine recommendation after pressure from families citing vaccine safety concerns largely based on powerful but unsubstantiated claims. All these instances illustrate shifts in and challenges to public confidence in vaccines.

Vaccine acceptance (or hesitancy) is influenced by an individual's knowledge about and previous experience with vaccine-preventable diseases; beliefs and practices among one's social circle; and sociopolitical factors, including the role and effectiveness of the public health system in a region's health care delivery. Both the World Health Organization Strategic Advisory Group of Experts on Immunization (SAGE) and the US National Vaccine Advisory Committee (NVAC, part of the Centers for Disease Control and Prevention) have convened working groups on vaccine hesitancy. Other countries have also focused on better understanding vaccine hesitancy, and since 2000, the number of published articles on this topic has increased fourfold.

What is vaccine hesitancy?

There is no simple answer to this question. In its publication, *The State of Vaccine Confidence*, the SAGE working group defines vaccine hesitancy as

> a behavior influenced by a number of factors including issues of confidence, complacency, and convenience. Vaccine-hesitant individuals are a heterogeneous group who hold varying degrees of indecision about specific vaccines or vaccination in general. Vaccine-hesitant individuals may accept all vaccines but remain concerned about vaccines; some may refuse or delay some vaccines, but accept others; some individuals may refuse all vaccines.

What is particularly striking about this definition is the broad range of motivations associated with hesitancy. A parent may be supportive of vaccines in general but may not prioritize vaccinating his or her child because of perceived low risk of vaccine-preventable diseases or because the cost of getting the child vaccinated is too high. Each of these domains is also influenced by other mitigating factors, including the beliefs and actions of family or friends, exposure to messages about vaccines through popular media, and previous experiences with the health care system. In other words, vaccine hesitancy is extraordinarily complex, and the different permutations of factors that influence hesitancy will differ by individual and region. In fact, a review of more than 1,000 studies on vaccine hesitancy could not identify one universal definition. Rather, the core of hesitancy is a "vaccine confidence gap."

What is meant by the "vaccine confidence gap"?

The vaccine confidence gap refers to eroding trust in vaccines and in immunization delivery systems. The SAGE working group defined *vaccine confidence* as trust in vaccine safety and effectiveness, the health care system that delivers vaccines, and the motivations of policymakers. When trust in any of these domains falters, a confidence gap can drive hesitancy.

How does vaccine hesitancy manifest?

No single trait, belief, or behavior is singularly associated with vaccine hesitancy. It is a continuum of beliefs and behaviors ranging from refusal of all vaccines to refusal of some vaccines to having questions about vaccines but still accepting recommendations.

It is important to note again that not all individuals who demonstrate vaccine hesitancy have a negative view of vaccines. Using the SAGE definition of hesitancy, individuals are just as likely to be hesitant due to sentiments such as complacency ("I am not worried about getting a vaccine-preventable disease"), convenience ("I didn't schedule an immunization visit because clinic hours do not work for my schedule"), or confidence ("I am delaying certain vaccines for my kids because I am worried about vaccine side effects"). These same individuals may also have questions that they would like to have answered about a vaccine before they accept a recommendation.

What is the difference between vaccine hesitancy and the anti-vaccine movement?

Vaccine hesitancy is a behavior demonstrated by an individual, sometimes quite passively. The anti-vaccination movement is a more activist group of individuals who *actively oppose* vaccination. In the United States, the anti-vaccine movement gained traction in the 1980s with a public outcry surrounding the whole cell diphtheria, tetanus, and pertussis vaccine (DTP). Because early pertussis vaccines were made from a whole killed pertussis bacteria, the vaccines carried a large number of antigens from the killed bacteria, producing a robust immune response. Some of the antigens stimulated an immune response in the nervous system. This led to various side effects, including higher fevers, prolonged crying episodes, and, in some cases, encephalopathy, which is a term referring to any change in brain function. Although these events would self-resolve, they also resulted in distress for families and concerns about potential long-term neurologic effects. These concerns became well-publicized in a 1982 news feature titled "DPT: Vaccine Roulette" that aired on major news network. The feature alleged that DTP caused brain damage and was unnecessarily dangerous. More significantly, it provided a mainstream media platform for the belief that the safety of vaccines is not guaranteed. This sparked the establishment of Dissatisfied Parents Together, which in 1991 became the National Vaccine Information Center, perhaps today's most vocal skeptic of vaccine safety and the current immunization program.

Why is it important to define vaccine hesitancy as a spectrum of beliefs?

Understanding the heterogeneity of vaccine hesitancy is important because such an understanding can help identify effective strategies to address it; one approach will not work for every person. Presuming that the ultimate goal is to improve trust in vaccines and overall acceptance, different approaches are likely needed for different individuals.

How common is vaccine hesitancy?

Although there has been an increased focus on vaccine hesitancy in recent years, the majority of individuals have an overall positive view of vaccines. According to a 2015 Gallup poll in the United States, nearly 80% of respondents believe that vaccination is "very" or "extremely" important.

However, even those with positive views may have questions or concerns regarding vaccine safety, how well vaccines work, the necessity of vaccines (especially when disease incidence is low), or the number of vaccines given at one time. The same Gallup poll found that 9% of respondents believe that vaccines are more dangerous than the diseases that they prevent, an increase from 6% in 2001. In addition, recent surveys of US pediatricians found that the vast majority (approximately 90%) received at least one vaccine refusal or request to delay a vaccine from parents per month. Among children from a multistate surveillance network who had not received at least one recommended vaccine for their age, an estimated 13% were undervaccinated due to parental choice to delay or refuse a vaccine. A very small proportion of parents, less than 5%, refuse all vaccines.

How is vaccine hesitancy measured?

It is relatively easy to report how frequently parents request to delay or refuse a vaccine; it is more difficult to identify the motivation and beliefs that underlie such requests. Some of this can be captured via surveys asking different questions about attitudes and beliefs related to vaccines or in-depth interviews to learn more about what might influence attitudes and beliefs about vaccines. There are also newly developed tools that ask a set of questions about vaccine-related beliefs that can predict who may be more likely to delay or refuse a vaccine. However, such tools have not yet been widely used in practice to produce actionable conclusions.

Perhaps more innovatively, research efforts are underway to monitor media and social media for emerging issues that might affect public sentiment about vaccines. Similar approaches have been used effectively to search for signs of emerging infectious diseases.

Which individuals may be more or less likely to be vaccine hesitant?

There is no "type" when it comes to vaccine-hesitant individuals. The multitude of individual traits at play (socioeconomic, health beliefs, etc.), combined with the many ways vaccine hesitancy can manifest behaviorally, defy simple generalizations of type.

A correlation has emerged, however, between vaccine hesitancy and scientific denialism—the rejection of a fact for which there is well-established scientific consensus. An example is the belief that HIV does not cause AIDS and instead is a claim created by scientists to deceive the public. Such beliefs may be backed by individuals who claim to be experts but at their heart go against well-established knowledge by advocating information that is not supported by reliable facts. Even without scientific denialism, trusting the reliability of information and distinguishing between facts and misinformation has become increasingly challenging, particularly in the wake of the 2016 US presidential election during which terms such as "alternative facts" and "fake news" emerged in an effort to delegitimize mainstream news reporting.

Are health care providers ever vaccine hesitant?

It is rare, but yes. The recommended immunization schedule is endorsed by nearly every professional organization for physicians, nurses, and allied health professionals. However, this does not mean that health care providers cannot have their own beliefs about vaccines—and sometimes their personal beliefs can influence the strength of their endorsement.

Provider recommendation for the HPV vaccine is an example of how provider hesitancy might occur. Because HPV is a sexually transmitted infection, some providers may not feel comfortable talking about sex with young or adolescent patients, or they may not think that their patients need the HPV vaccine until they are older. These beliefs are well-documented reasons why certain providers may not recommend HPV vaccines, especially to the 11- and 12-year-old age group targeted in the routine recommendation. For the most part, however, providers who may be hesitant about HPV vaccines generally endorse and strongly recommend all the other routinely recommended vaccines.

There is a much smaller group of health care providers who are hesitant about all vaccines. One board-certified pediatrician in California has published a book recommending an alternative vaccine schedule that spreads out and delays routinely recommended vaccines, and this publication has found a following among some parents in the United States. His schedule is based on concerns about vaccine safety, especially about exposure to aluminum in vaccines. His book also notably downplays the risk of vaccine-preventable diseases and suggests that some vaccines are not necessary because of herd immunity. Many of its claims are unsubstantiated and even contradict well-established evidence.

What are the implications of vaccine hesitancy?

When vaccine hesitancy prompts individuals to delay or forego receipt of certain vaccines, it produces a higher number of individuals in a community who are susceptible, or at risk,

for a vaccine-preventable disease. Also, when these immunization rates drop below levels needed to prevent disease transmission (i.e., the level needed to achieve herd immunity), these
diseases return, especially when unvaccinated individuals live
in close proximity within a community. Recent years have seen
significant increases in the incidences of pertussis and other
vaccine-preventable diseases, such as measles. Studies on these
outbreaks have shown an association between the proportion
of children with exemptions to school-entry requirements and
the incidence of these preventable diseases.

As an illustration, a review of 32 published reports of pertussis outbreaks over 40 years found that the risk for pertussis
was 6–20 times higher among children with an exemption to
school-entry vaccine requirements compared to children who
were fully vaccinated. In one-fourth of these outbreaks, 60–90%
of the pertussis cases were voluntarily unvaccinated or undervaccinated. In pertussis outbreaks in California and Michigan,
census tracts with higher exemption rates were more likely to
be within a cluster of pertussis occurrence.

The association between school exemptions and pertussis outbreaks also demonstrates the impact that state vaccine
policies can have on hesitancy and, subsequently, immunization rates. The ease of obtaining an exemption to school entry
requirements, in tandem with the availability of personal belief
exemptions, increases the likelihood of incidence of pertussis
in any given community.

What are the practical and economic costs associated with disease outbreaks that result from vaccine hesitancy?

A disease outbreak yields significant costs—financial and
otherwise—for affected individuals, families, and communities. When a child or adult develops a vaccine-preventable
disease, the illness may require a visit to an emergency room
or health care provider, medications, and hospitalization, and
it may result in lost productivity from missing work. Some

vaccine-preventable diseases, such as meningococcus, can lead to permanent medical problems (e.g., deafness or limb amputation). Recent analyses have estimated that the costs associated with medical care during a whooping cough outbreak are $181 for each affected adult and $2,822 for each affected infant. For meningococcal disease, medical costs can reach more than $200,000 per individual.

In addition to the individual costs of medical care, an outbreak requires intervention from public health authorities to investigate the outbreak and take measures to stop it. This may include identifying all of the contacts of an infected individual to search for additional cases, performing diagnostic tests, and distributing vaccines. Depending on the size and location of the outbreak, public health costs can range from approximately $10,000 to several million dollars. Who covers these costs? It is largely public health departments that often do not have a budget for unexpected events such as outbreaks. (For context, only 0.5% of the 2014 fiscal year federal health care budget was earmarked for public health activities.)

How can vaccine hesitancy be addressed?

Concerns about vaccines are likely to persist and increase as the immunization schedule continues to evolve. To combat this, the scientific and medical establishments are charged with finding effective strategies to address the reasons underlying hesitancy ("barriers to vaccination"), as well as factors that may drive vaccine acceptance ("facilitators of vaccination"). A considerable amount of this chapter has focused on exploring barriers. But what about facilitators that increase vaccination? For the most part, these factors are related to convenience, confidence, and complacency and will include access, trust, awareness, and motivation. Targeting each of these areas demands a different approach.

Communication about vaccines that can address concerns or raise awareness about recommendations is an imperative.

However, in the age of immediate access to information—and in an environment such as the Internet in which all information is treated as equal—the way in which information is communicated is as important as the content itself. Individuals' decisions related to health hinge not just on knowledge but also on how they think and feel about the action; the content of the scientific community's message is only a small part of the battle. Studies have shown that giving parents a description or photo of a child with measles increased knowledge about measles but also increased beliefs that the measles vaccine causes side effects (as opposed to increasing beliefs about the need for vaccination). A review of 23 studies evaluating the effectiveness of different parent-focused educational materials found that only approximately half resulted in improved attitudes toward vaccination or greater intention to vaccinate. The overwhelming takeaway in studies such as these is that the way information is communicated does matter—arguably as much as the content itself.

Health care providers remain the paramount source of information for individuals seeking to learn more about vaccines: A strong recommendation from a health care provider is associated with an increased likelihood of getting vaccinated. Health care providers may also be better able to tailor their messages to specific concerns or follow-up for ongoing questions. Communication to individuals may also occur through public education and awareness efforts, which broadly disseminate messages about vaccines or vaccine-preventable diseases. For these campaigns to be effective, messages need to be relevant and compelling, especially because there is so much competing inaccurate information available about vaccines that may be equally compelling.

Where do people get information about vaccines?

Health care providers are often cited as the preferred source of vaccine information, but an increasing proportion of individuals use the Internet as their primary source of health information, including 42% who consult the Internet specifically for vaccine information. In considering these statistics, it is important to note that three-fourths of users trust information found on the Internet and only sometimes or never evaluate the reliability of information from websites. A substantial proportion of people also rely on their social networks for information about vaccines, which means that social media has become a primary information source for information on vaccines and medicine. This is bad news for the scientific establishment: Approximately one-third of YouTube videos about vaccines have negative messages about them, and approximately one-half disseminate inaccurate information.

Vaccines have also become more prominent in popular media coverage. The news feature "DTP: Vaccine Roulette" aired on a major news network in 1982, and since that time, stories related to vaccine safety concerns have continued to make headlines—many opinion-driven—across major news outlets. Relatively recently, vaccines have also entered political discourse. In two recent elections, candidates have directly discussed vaccines, sometimes broadcasting inaccurate information on highly public platforms, including presidential debates. Vaccines remain a galvanizing policy issue and will likely remain so for the foreseeable future.

What are the most reliable sources of information related to vaccines?

This is the question that is most commonly mitigated by an individual's preexisting beliefs. Generally, with regard to vaccination, health care providers are considered a reliable source of information. In one nationally representative survey, 82% of parents stated that they rely on their child's health care provider for information. However, as detailed previously, individuals also heavily rely on the Internet for health information. Performing a Google search about vaccines will most likely

Table 8.1 Websites That Provide Reliable Information About Vaccines, Immunization Recommendations, and Vaccine Policy

Organization	Website
Immunization Action Coalition	www.immunize.org
Parents of Kids with Infectious Diseases	www.pkids.org
Voices for Vaccines	www.voicesforvaccines.org
Vaccine Education Center	www.vaccine.chop.edu
Every Child by Two	www.ecbt.org

lead to a wide array of websites and blogs, many of which will communicate misinformation and sometimes very strong anti-vaccine messages. Table 8.1 provides a list of websites that provide reliable information about vaccines, immunization recommendations, and vaccine policy from the perspective of health care providers, public health officials, and parents.

How can one evaluate the reliability of information?

The evolving media landscape offers a readily accessible platform for every perspective and opinion—a challenge when one is searching for authoritative information on a medical or scientific topic.

When evaluating the reliability of information, it is important to consider source, tone, and content. Because essentially any individual or organization can write a report, a key first step is to read about the presenter, his or her expertise, and the presentation's stated goals; in aggregate, these factors speak to reliability of the source. Websites should be upfront about their purpose and intended audience while also providing clear information about sponsorship, membership, and site content and privacy policy. Sites should also offer a description of the process used to select their site content, including some kind of review process. References should be provided for medical claims.

Is the information based on a scientific study or anecdote? Personal stories can be a compelling way to share experiences, but if you are trying to determine whether a vaccine is associated with a potential side effect, a story will not provide the answer: The report should include information from a scientific study and give some details about how the study was done. In addition, the way in which information is presented is important; there should be a focus on specific facts rather than opinion or inference. This can be difficult to disentangle because information is often presented with a spin based on the author's perspective.

Last, when evaluating scientific studies for conclusions or facts, remember that not all scientific studies are good studies. A study is based on statistics that measure whether a significant association between an intervention or exposure and an outcome exists. To do this well, a study needs to be large enough to find an association, there needs to be a comparison (control) group, and the study's methods need to account for other factors that might bias or confuse an association. The strongest studies use randomization—people are randomly placed into the exposure and control groups to help minimize bias. Reliable study results are also supported by other studies in which similar results are obtained by others who have examined the same association in different groups of people. This is an important test of validity.

9

ON THE HORIZON

Despite the challenges of increasing vaccine hesitancy among the public, vaccines remain one of society's most important and influential tools for promoting public health. Accordingly, the immunization schedule will continue to evolve and expand in response to ongoing shifts in the diseases that threaten us, including emerging infectious diseases. The ongoing importance of vaccines is reflected in the public and private investment that continues to be poured into research: 2011–2020 has been termed the "Decade of Vaccines" by the World Health Organization (WHO), and unprecedented investments in development and infrastructure ensure that the benefits of vaccines are being optimized and made accessible worldwide. What can we expect?

What new vaccines are under development?

According to a 2016 report by WHO, approximately 600 vaccine candidates targeting 110 pathogens are under development. Some of these are new formulations of existing, licensed vaccines, but many are for diseases for which no vaccine exists. Some of these new vaccine candidates target not only infectious diseases but also conditions such as certain cancers, which until recently were not preventable. Given the significant investments required to develop and produce a vaccine, current research and development are guided by disease burden and the promise of the vaccine candidate to prevent disease. Particular effort and resources are being dedicated to developing vaccines for the following:

- Respiratory syncytial virus (RSV) and group B streptococcus (GBS) for pregnant women
- Universal influenza vaccine that would not need to be changed each year
- Malaria and tuberculosis
- Human immunodeficiency virus (HIV)
- Group A streptococcus
- Emerging infections such as Ebola virus and Zika virus

Vaccines during pregnancy

Why are group B streptococcus and respiratory syncytial virus vaccines being developed for pregnant women?

GBS and RSV are two of the most common causes of severe illness in newborns and infants. GBS is a leading cause of meningitis and bloodstream infections, whereas RSV can cause severe pneumonia. Risk for these infections is highest in the first few months of life, so vaccinating pregnant mothers (as is the current practice with pertussis vaccines, or Tdap, for example) helps the mother produce protective antibodies that are passed to her developing infant, protecting the infant from the time of delivery. For GBS, vaccination may also reduce the likelihood that the mother will become infected herself and expose the infant. Because many women carry GBS in their bodies, especially in the birth canal, some infants can be exposed to the bacteria during the birth process. Protocols are in place to prevent this from happening (women are tested during pregnancy and receive antibiotics if positive), but they do not prevent all transmission, and exposure can also happen after delivery. A vaccine for pregnant women represents an opportunity to stop infections before they occur.

What are the challenges to developing vaccines for pregnant women?

Although the use of pertussis (Tdap) and influenza vaccines during pregnancy has become standard practice, physicians remain hesitant to recommend any pharmaceutical product to pregnant patients unless the product has been rigorously tested for safety. As described in Chapter 5, safety is rigorously evaluated during vaccine development and after licensure, but vaccine clinical trials have not traditionally included pregnant women. This is changing for current vaccines under development for pregnant women, which would face two phases of clinical trials: first, studies in healthy, nonpregnant women of childbearing age to establish safety and then studies in pregnant women.

Another question concerning vaccines for pregnant women is whether these vaccines would be included in the National Vaccine Injury Compensation Program, which covers vaccines routinely recommended for children. Because children also receive influenza and Tdap vaccines, the program extends to those vaccines even when given to pregnant women. However, the program would not extend to RSV and GBS if these vaccines were exclusively given to pregnant women. This issue was taken up by the Advisory Commission on Childhood Vaccines, which recommended that the US Secretary of Health and Human Services consider a pathway for inclusion of such vaccines in the program. This legislation was introduced and passed in 2016, providing a pathway for coverage.

Vaccines for emerging infectious diseases

Will we be ready for the next outbreak or pandemic for emerging infections such as Ebola and Zika viruses?

The Ebola virus epidemic in West Africa and the Zika virus in the Americas have served as a wake-up call for the need to strengthen vaccine development preparedness so that populations can survive in the face of new infectious diseases. WHO has identified 10 different viruses that are likely to cause an outbreak in the near future, including Ebola and Zika viruses. Early identification of threats is important for future outbreaks, especially considering the response to the 2014 West African Ebola crisis: Soon after the epidemic began, when it became clear that efforts to prevent transmission were not working, the push to develop a vaccine (a collaboration between academic institutions, WHO, and pharmaceutical companies) had a late start. By the time a vaccine candidate appeared to be effective, the epidemic was ending, and many people had already been affected.

Ebola was not a new virus when it struck West Africa, and extinguishing the outbreak could have been done more quickly had new vaccines been under development before the epidemic began. As a practical matter, this level of preparation was extremely challenging: The steps involved in vaccine development were too numerous, too rigid, and too uncoordinated across countries. In the case of Ebola, it was especially challenging because affected regions lacked the resources to sponsor vaccine development.

In response, the Coalition for Epidemic Preparedness Innovations was established in January 2016. The coalition is a public–private cooperative encompassing 80 organizations and 200 individuals to coordinate vaccine development against epidemic infectious diseases—especially diseases that may arise in countries that would not be able to afford purchasing vaccines. With a budget of $1 billion for 5 years (most of it coming from national governments and private donors such as the Gates Foundation), the coalition aims to advance candidate vaccines for two or three priority diseases through the first phases of clinical development. By doing so, the coalition will ready the candidate vaccines for efficacy trials in the event of an epidemic or pandemic, thereby speeding the response. The coalition's work will also include support for ushering candidates through the regulatory process and establishing international stockpiles so that new vaccines can be quickly delivered to regions most affected by an outbreak.

Will there be a new vaccine for Zika virus?

In August 2015, an increased number of infants born with microcephaly, or abnormal brain development, were reported in Brazil. In November 2015, the Brazilian Ministry of Health announced an association between microcephaly and infection with the mosquito-borne Zika virus during pregnancy. Zika virus was first identified in Brazil in April 2015, and since that time, it has rapidly spread across South and Central America, the Caribbean, and pockets of the southern United States. Although the majority of Zika virus infections do not result in congenital problems, the association between Zika virus infection and abnormal brain development in infants constitutes an unprecedented public health emergency. As the virus has spread, so has the push to develop a vaccine.

The need for a vaccine is amplified by the inadequacy of other prevention strategies: People become infected if they are bitten by an infected mosquito, but there have also been documented instances of transmission through sexual contact, with the virus appearing to remain active in some bodily fluids (including semen) for several months after initial infection. Although public health services are experienced in installing measures to control mosquito-borne illnesses, these strategies will not be as effective with a fast-traveling, long-lasting, multivector infection such as Zika.

Encouragingly for scientists, Zika viruses are similar to other mosquito-borne viruses for which effective vaccines already exist. This provides a blueprint for starting Zika virus vaccine development. What will be more challenging is ensuring that a Zika vaccine works well—and deciding who needs to be vaccinated to provide protection when the risk for severe outcomes is highest. To prevent Zika's congenital problems in fetuses, pregnant women may need to be the target group for vaccination; however, they would require vaccination early in pregnancy because the highest risk for microcephaly appears to be associated with infections that occur in the first or early second trimester. Complicating matters further, many women do not know they are pregnant until well into their first trimester, and by then it may be too late to induce an adequate immune response to provide protection. There is also the baseline challenge of developing vaccines for pregnant women, which requires a longer timeline to conduct trials in both nonpregnant adults and pregnant women to confirm vaccine safety and efficacy.

An alternate strategy would be to develop a Zika vaccine for nonpregnant women of childbearing age and men to provide protection before pregnancy. A vaccine could also be developed for children, similar to the strategy used to prevent congenital problems from rubella. The success of either of these strategies, however, is contingent upon developing a vaccine that can spark long-lasting immunity to the Zika virus.

Whatever the strategy, vaccine development must occur first, and that development must balance urgency with the steps necessary for vaccine safety and efficacy. Currently, several vaccine candidates have successfully led to good immune responses in animal models, but only three have moved to Phase I safety trials and one moved to Phase II clinical trials in March 2017.

Preparing for the next influenza pandemic

What is the difference between an epidemic and a pandemic?

Epidemics and pandemics are both types of large outbreaks. An *epidemic* refers to a widespread incidence of an infectious disease in a community or local region. A *pandemic* refers to an epidemic over a larger geographic area. Either type of outbreak can occur when a new pathogen is introduced to a community: Because there are no immune individuals, everyone is susceptible.

Influenza is an excellent example. It is a virus that changes every year, and usually the changes are minor enough that some people will have immunity held over from previous influenza infection or vaccination. However, the annual changes in influenza are enough to bring about new infections (a dynamic known as *antigenic drift*), necessitating a new influenza vaccine every year to match the circulating viruses. Sometimes a more significant change occurs, which is called *antigenic shift*.

A recent example of antigenic shift is the 2009 novel influenza A H1N1 virus that launched a global influenza pandemic. Here, we saw the arrival of a new influenza type that first emerged in April 2009, and by May 2009, it had spread throughout the world. Because this was a new influenza type, people had no immunity from previous infection or vaccination and were more likely to get sick if exposed to the virus. This led to rapid proliferation—many infected people spreading virus to many susceptible people. Because the 2009 H1N1 strain affected multiple countries throughout the world, it was termed a pandemic. Influenza causes epidemics every year due to antigenic drift, and it causes pandemics every few decades due to antigenic shift.

How does antigenic drift and shift occur? Why does this not occur with other viruses or bacteria?

Viruses and bacteria do what they can to increase their chances for survival. Because they are so small and have fairly simple genetic material, they reproduce quickly and can also make small mutations or changes that can help them survive. Thus, for influenza, when it causes an infection, people make antibodies to kill the virus. The virus will then try to change so that these antibodies do not recognize it as well. Humans make antibodies that latch to two different parts of the influenza virus' surface: hemaglutinin and neuraminidase. This is also the part of the virus that can change fairly easily. For this reason, investigators are working to identify new ways to make influenza vaccines that do not depend on these ever-changing surface proteins.

New influenza strains also occur when genes from two different influenza types mix together, especially when one is human and the other is from an animal. Usually, the types of influenza that infect animals do not know how to survive in humans, but in rare cases when the genes do combine, the virus can learn this new skill. This is one of the reasons why public health officials monitor avian or bird flu so closely.

Are we getting any closer to an influenza vaccine that does not have to be changed every year?

Significant resources and focus have been devoted to influenza vaccine development, particularly improvements to the vaccine's production and effectiveness. Development of a universal influenza vaccine is high on this priority list as well, but it has proven challenging. A universal vaccine will require the ability to identify a part of the virus that does not change and also sparks a good enough antibody response to provide protection. Some vaccine candidates are focusing on a different part of the hemaglutinin protein: Current vaccines use the top, or head, of the protein, whereas the newer candidate vaccines use the more stable stalk. Other vaccine candidates focus on different virus proteins altogether, but these options would only make infection less severe, not prevent infection entirely. Last, some vaccine candidates use a helper substance, or adjuvant, that helps boost the antibody response for a wider range of proteins that may be shared across different influenza strains. These new possibilities may mean that a new vaccine would not be needed every year, but most of these vaccine candidates are still in the preclinical or early clinical trial phases.

Another focus for influenza vaccine development is speed— finding a way to manufacture more vaccine, faster. The current vaccine's dependence on eggs for vaccine production has made it difficult to scale-up production when need is greatest, especially in lower income countries. Some new vaccines do not require the use of eggs to grow influenza virus; these are known as cell-culture influenza vaccines.

Human Immunodeficiency Virus Vaccines

Are we getting closer to a vaccine to prevent human immunodeficiency virus?

According to WHO, an estimated 35.3 million people are infected with HIV worldwide. Although the development of effective medicines has greatly improved associated illness and survival after infection, there are still more than 1.5 million deaths per year and an estimated 6,300 new infections per day, primarily in low- and middle-income countries with lack of access to health care and medicines. New HIV infections have also persisted or increased among certain groups in the United States, including young adults. This suggests that existing prevention strategies have not maintained their ability to substantially reduce infection rates, highlighting the call for vaccine development as a potential solution.

However, during the more than 30 years since HIV vaccine development began, an effective vaccine has yet to be developed. Thirty vaccine candidates have been tested in more than 85 trials, but none of them have passed vetting for efficacy. The closest vaccine candidate was RV144, which in 2009 was found to have an efficacy of only 31.2%. This was not sufficient to move forward with production, but it did provide a good foundation for new candidates.

Why has it been so challenging to make an HIV vaccine? This is mostly attributable to the virus itself. HIV is a diverse virus that frequently mutates, making it difficult for scientists to identify one stable target for a vaccine. HIV is also known to be elusive, avoiding the immune system and hiding out in different organ systems, making it difficult to determine which part of the virus could be targeted to spark an immune response. Recent shifts in scientific research have also brought a reduction in funding for HIV vaccine development, making it difficult to maintain momentum.

As HIV vaccine development continues, new approaches remain under investigation. The results are mixed: Since RV144 in 2009, no candidate vaccines have reached Phase II or III clinical trials.

Therapeutic vaccines

Are vaccines being developed that can treat
rather than prevent illnesses?

Vaccines are generally thought of as a prevention tool, but for some conditions, their ability to spark an immune response could be used as treatment. Cancer is a good example. Therapeutic (as opposed to prophylactic or preventative) vaccines work by producing immune cells that can target certain markers on the outside of tumor cells. During cancer, certain cells in the body gain a mutation that makes them grow out of control, but all of the cells look alike and may have tumor-specific proteins on the outside that mark them as abnormal; these proteins could be targeted with a vaccine, especially during the early stages of cancer. Such vaccines can either slow down or stop cancer cell growth, kill cancer cells that have not been removed by other treatments, or prevent recurrence of cancer. Although the science of this approach sounds promising, it has been challenging to achieve—mostly because some of the proteins produced by cancer cells look too much like regular cell proteins. Cancer cells are also adept at avoiding the immune system, sometimes by changing their cancer proteins just enough so that they will not be recognized. For these reasons, relatively few therapeutic cancer vaccines gain approval by the US Food and Drug Administration (FDA). The first cancer treatment vaccine was approved in 2010 for metastatic prostate cancer after use of the vaccine was shown to increase survival by an average of 4 months. In 2015, the FDA approved a vaccine for metastatic melanoma that cannot be removed surgically. Although these are the only two approved therapeutic cancer vaccines, several others are under investigation, including therapies for breast, kidney, lung, and other cancers.

There are also two approved and recommended vaccines that prevent cancer: the hepatitis B and the HPV vaccines. Each of these viruses is a known cause of cancer (liver cancer for hepatitis B, and anal, genital, throat, and cervical cancers for HPV).

In addition to vaccines for cancer therapy, other therapeutic vaccines against tobacco addiction are under development. These vaccines work by producing antibodies against nicotine; the antibodies attach to nicotine circulating in the blood and keep it from attaching to receptors in the brain—the trigger for addiction. Currently, however, only one vaccine candidate has advanced through Phase III clinical trials, and it was not found to be effective.

Disease elimination and eradication

Vaccine introduction and widespread implementation of immunization programs has resulted in the elimination or near elimination of several vaccine-preventable diseases. Although eradication is not a likely endpoint for many vaccine-preventable diseases, it is achievable for some. Most notably, significant effort is being expended to eradicate polio. It is quite a challenge to eliminate or completely eradicate a disease that regularly circulates, or is endemic, in a region.

What is an endemic disease?

An endemic disease is one that enjoys sustained transmission in a community. In the United States, diseases such as measles and polio have been eliminated, meaning there is no longer any sustained transmission between one person and another.

These diseases may still arise in isolated cases, but because almost everyone else is immune, the pathogen has nowhere to go and it dies out. When cases surface, the pathogen has typically been introduced from somewhere else. If transmission is able to occur regularly—that is, the pathogen always has a place to go and survive—it becomes endemic, which means that it belongs to a particular people or country.

How do we achieve elimination or eradication of infectious diseases?

Elimination of an infectious disease means that there are no more new cases of a disease within a specific area. Because the infectious disease may still exist elsewhere—that is, it can be imported—elimination also requires ongoing efforts to prevent the pathogen from re-emerging. This can generally be achieved by maintaining sufficient immunization rates to prevent transmission when the pathogen is introduced. Thus, for example, if a person with measles visits a community but everyone else in the community is immunized and therefore not susceptible, no new cases will develop. Measles and polio are both examples of infectious diseases that have been eliminated from the United States but still circulate in other countries.

Eradication refers to a permanent elimination of an infectious disease worldwide. There are no new cases anywhere, so no interventions such as ongoing immunization are required. Smallpox is an example of an eradicated disease. There is also a global initiative to eradicate polio, which is in the final phases of implementation.

One could argue that elimination or eradication is the ultimate goal of disease control efforts, and vaccination is the primary tool in either pursuit. However, there are a few other factors that are necessary for elimination or eradication to be feasible. First, the pathogen must only infect humans; if the virus or bacteria also lives in animals or the environment, it becomes very difficult to control ongoing exposure via animal-to-human or water-to-human transmission. It also helps to have a vaccine that prevents not only active infection but also carriage or asymptomatic infection—pathogens can be passed to others even if they do not manifest in illness symptoms. Finally, it is important to have a reliable way to identify the infection in the first place so that other disease-control strategies can be paired with vaccines to minimize disease impact.

What is the Global Polio Eradication Initiative?

The Global Polio Eradication Initiative was launched in 1988, when 350,000 cases of paralytic polio were reported worldwide. (In comparison, in 2015, only 70 cases were reported, all of them in two countries.) Why was the initiative established and how did it achieve this success? Until a vaccine was introduced in the 1950s, polio was a devastating disease that affected children in developed and developing countries. Although the majority of infected children were asymptomatic when infected, 1 in 200 developed paralysis. In 1952, just before the vaccine's introduction in the United States, 58,000 cases of paralytic polio were documented, accounting for 3,145 deaths and 22,000 children with permanent disability.

Polio infects the gastrointestinal tract, which means that infected individuals shed the virus through their stool. Accordingly, exposure to polio frequently stems from contact with contaminated surfaces or water. The two types of polio vaccines (an inactivated virus vaccine, which protects against two virus types, and the oral vaccine, which protects against all three virus types) both prevent infection, but some countries struggled to achieve elimination due to poor sanitation—itself a thorny problem, one arguably larger in scale than vaccination. So even as rates of polio decreased significantly, work remained to be done.

The Global Eradication Initiative is led by WHO, UNICEF, Rotary International, the US Centers for Disease Control and

Prevention, and the Gates Foundation. The Initiative's initial goal was to eradicate polio by 2000 through efforts to increase immunization rates and access in affected areas. Polio was eliminated from the Americas in 1993 and the Western Pacific in 1997, but slow progress from 2000 until 2010 resulted in 1,352 cases reported in 20 countries. By 2016, there were only 35 cases reported, all centered in Afghanistan, Pakistan, and Nigeria. (Africa was actually polio-free as of 2014, but the reported cases in Nigeria in 2016 ended this streak.) Eradication is close, but challenges remain.

Insecurity from armed conflict is one major barrier to achieving eradication, as militant groups in some countries often prevent children from gaining access to immunization services. This challenge has been overcome to some degree through negotiation (via local partners) with opposition groups, including Boko Haram in Nigeria. Other militant groups have installed systematic resistance to vaccination. This has been especially disruptive in Pakistan, where the Taliban openly banned polio vaccination and promoted violence against vaccinators. In response, the Global Eradication Initiative has worked with Islamic groups to disseminate information to advocate for polio vaccination, with some success.

Another persisting barrier to polio eradication has been the circulation of the vaccine-related poliovirus. The oral polio vaccine (OPV) is a live virus vaccine that in rare instances (1 in 2.7 million children) can mutate enough in the gut to cause paralytic polio. In communities in which vaccination rates are low, children who receive OPV can shed the vaccine virus in their stool, potentially spreading it to others. Although this happens infrequently, it poses a challenge to full eradication. With so few reported cases globally, countries have added inactivated viral vaccines to their schedules in 2016. The inactivated vaccine is injected, not oral, so it results in less shedding in the stool and no opportunity for a live virus to mutate and cause infection. All OPVs will be removed from circulation after 2020 if there is no more wild polio virus transmission in Afghanistan, Pakistan, or Nigeria. With this final push, it may be possible to achieve complete eradication, but a risk of resurgence remains if vaccination rates do not remain high. If all countries and regions do not detect polio cases for 3 years, the world will be declared polio-free.

Can we expect eradication or near eradication of any other vaccine-preventable diseases in the next 20 years?

Measles eradication has been cited as a potential public health goal. The number of cases has significantly decreased since vaccine introduction, but the disease remains a leading cause of death worldwide among children younger than age 5 years. In 2014, an estimated 114,000 cases of measles occurred. Some countries with well-established immunization programs have had substantial outbreaks, including more than 37,000 cases in the European Union in 2011. Even in the United States, where in 2000 measles was declared eliminated, new outbreaks have occurred, often initiated by travelers returning from regions with endemic measles.

Thus, although measles fulfills many of the criteria for eradication, challenges remain. Measles only occurs in and is spread between people, which means that blocking its transmission between individuals will effectively eliminate the virus' reservoir and ability to spread. The virus is also reliably diagnosed based on symptomatic manifestations and blood tests. Herd immunity for measles would require vaccination rates of at least 95%; this is achievable but requires ongoing attention and public vigilance, which is no small task. In the United States in 2015, measles vaccine rates among 19- to 35-month-old children in most US states were greater than 90%, but only 11 states had rates greater than 95%. And the majority of people affected by measles outbreaks in the United States are unvaccinated by choice.

APPENDIX

Schedules and Overviews for Common Child and Adolescent Vaccines

Vaccine	Vaccine-Preventable Disease	Brief History	Current Routine Schedule (United States)	Reported Adverse Events[a,b]	Vaccine Effectiveness
Hepatitis B (HepB) Recombinant vaccine	Hepatitis B Virus transmitted through blood and other body fluids; can also be transmitted from mother to infant Causes acute and chronic liver disease. Chronic infection can lead to liver failure, cirrhosis, or cancer (causes 50% of hepatocellular cancer).	Before vaccine introduction ~18,000 children <10 years old infected each year Since vaccine introduction 2,895 cases reported in 2012 90% of infected infants develop chronic infection.	1st dose: birth 2nd dose: 1–2 months 3rd dose: 6–18 months After birth, may be given as part of a combination vaccine (DTaP–HepB–IPV) at 2, 4, and 6 months	Pain or soreness at the injection site, mild fever, headache, fatigue	>90% protection to infants, children, and adults immunized with 3-dose series before exposure to the virus. Some people may not respond to first series and will require a second series.
Rotavirus (RV1 and RV5) Oral live attenuated virus vaccine	Rotavirus Virus that infects the lining of the intestines and causes diarrhea and sometimes vomiting; can lead to severe dehydration Spread through fecal–oral route	Before vaccine introduction 2.7 million children affected every year. Almost every child had a rotavirus infection by age 5 years. Since vaccine introduction 40,000–50,000 fewer rotavirus hospitalizations per year since 2008	1st dose: 2 months 2nd dose: 4 months 3rd dose: 6 months RV1 is 2-dose series RV5 is 3-dose series	Vomiting, diarrhea, irritability, fever	Approximately 9 out of 10 vaccinated children are protected from severe rotavirus illness, whereas 7 out of 10 children will be protected from rotavirus infection of any severity.

Vaccine	Pathogen	Before/Since vaccine introduction	Indicated for children	Adverse reactions	Notes
Diphtheria–tetanus–acellular Pertussis (DTaP) Protein subunit vaccine	*Corynebacterium diphtheriae* Bacteria that cause a throat infection that can lead to severe breathing problems, heart failure, paralysis, and death in 5–10% of cases. Severe infections due to a toxin made by the bacteria	Before vaccine introduction Diphtheria: 100,000–200,000 cases/year and 13,000–15,000 deaths/year Tetanus: 500–600 cases/year Pertussis: 175,000 reported cases/year	Indicated for children <7 years old 1st dose: 2 months 2nd dose: 4 months 3rd dose: 6 months 4th dose: 15–18 months 5th dose: 4–6 years May be given as part of a combination vaccine (DTaP–HepB–IPV) at 2, 4, and 6 months	Pain, redness or swelling at the injection site, low-grade fever, drowsiness. Local reaction more frequent after 4th or 5th dose—can have full arm/leg swelling that self-resolves	Among children completing 5-dose series, 98 out of 100 children are fully protected the year following the 5th dose. Immunity to pertussis begins to wane ~3–5 years after vaccination.
	Clostridium tetani (lockjaw) Bacteria that release a toxin that attacks the nervous system, causing muscles spasms and potentially death. Can cause infection in newborns if mother does not have immunity	Since vaccine introduction Diphtheria: 5 cases reported since 2000 in United States; outbreaks still occur globally Tetanus: ~30 cases/year, almost all among unvaccinated people or those who have not had a 10-year booster		Rare (<1 in 10,000 doses): high fever, seizure with fever, persistent crying	
	Bordetella pertussis (whopping cough) Bacteria that cause severe coughing spasms. Complications include pneumonia, seizures, brain damage, and death. Risk of complications highest in young infants	Pertussis: by 1980, <3,000 cases per year but now a resurgence (>48,000 cases in 2012)—related to waning immunity with the acellular pertussis vaccine and underimmunization			

(continued)

Vaccine	Vaccine-Preventable Disease	Brief History	Current Routine Schedule (United States)	Reported Adverse Events[a,b]	Vaccine Effectiveness
Haemophilus influenzae type b conjugate (Hib) Conjugate protein vaccine	*Haemophilus influenzae* type b Bacteria that cause pneumonia, bloodstream infections, meningitis, and infections of the bones and joints	Before vaccine introduction ~20,000 children <5 years with serious (or fatal) infections per year Since vaccine introduction 25 reported cases per year 2003–2010. Most cases among un- or undervaccinated children	1st dose: 2 months 2nd dose: 4 months 3rd dose: 6 months 4th dose: 12–15 months OR 3rd dose: 12–15 months[c]	Pain and soreness at injection site	95–100% effective at preventing serious infections after primary series
Pneumococcal Conjugate (PCV13) Conjugate protein vaccine	*Streptococcus pneumoniae* Bacteria that cause ear and sinus infections, pneumonia, bloodstream infections, and meningitis, especially in young children and older adults Current vaccine targets 13 serotypes (of ~90 total serotypes)	Before vaccine introduction 17,000 cases of invasive disease (bloodstream infections, meningitis) and 5 million cases of middle ear infection among children <5 years old Since vaccine introduction 99% reduction in invasive disease caused by vaccine serotypes in children <5 years old and 76% reduction in disease caused by all types. Significant decreases in older adults >65 years old due to herd immunity	1st dose: 2 months 2nd dose: 4 months 3rd dose: 6 months 4th dose: 12–15 months	Pain and swelling at the injection site, fever, high fever (>102°F), decreased appetite, irritability	97% reduction in invasive disease caused by vaccine types among children 75 out of 100 adults age 65 years or older protected against invasive pneumococcal disease

Vaccine	Disease	Schedule	Side effects	Effectiveness
Inactivated polio vaccine (IPV) Inactivated virus vaccine	Poliovirus Enterovirus that first infects the throat and lining of the intestines and then can invade an infected person's brain and spinal cord, causing paralysis (paralytic poliomyelitis)	Before the polio vaccine, 13,000–20,000 cases of paralytic polio per year. The United States has been polio-free since 1979; last imported case in 1993. Near eradication worldwide	1st dose: 2 months 2nd dose: 4 months 3rd dose: 6–18 months 4th dose: 4–6 years May be given as part of a combination vaccine (DTaP–HepB–IPV) at 2, 4, and 6 months	Redness and pain at injection site	> 90% immune after 2 doses; 99% immune after 3 doses
Influenza (IIV and LAIV) IIV—inactivated influenza virus vaccine LAIV—live attenuated influenza virus vaccine	Influenza virus Causes respiratory infections and pneumonia. Complications include secondary bacterial pneumonia, respiratory failure, and death. Circulating strains of influenza may change each year, which leads to almost yearly changes to the influenza vaccine.	Yearly epidemics—activity usually peaks December—March 200,000 hospitalizations per year. Highest hospitalization rates among young children, infants, and older adults	6–23 months: annual vaccination (IIV only) 1 or 2 doses 2–8 years: annual vaccination 1 or 2 doses (IIV or LAIV) 9 years and older: annual vaccination 1 dose only (IIV or LAIV)	Redness, soreness, or swelling at the injection site; muscle aches; headache; low-grade fever	Vaccine effectiveness varies by year. Generally reduces the risk of influenza by 50–60% when most circulating flu viruses are similar to vaccine viruses

(continued)

Vaccine	Vaccine-Preventable Disease	Brief History	Current Routine Schedule (United States)	Reported Adverse Events[a,b]	Vaccine Effectiveness
Measles, mumps, and rubella (MMR) Live attenuated virus vaccine	Measles virus Causes fever, rash, red eyes, and runny nose. Complications include encephalitis (1 in 1,000 cases) and death. Mumps virus Causes parotitis or swelling of the salivary glands, and orchitis (swelling of the testicles). Complications include meningitis and kidney problems. Rubella virus Causes fever; sore throat; rash; and red, itchy eyes. Pregnant women infected with rubella may suffer a miscarriage or the infant may have serious birth defects (ccongenital rubella syndrome).	Before vaccine introduction Measles: 500,000 reported cases per year Mumps: More than 160,000 reported cases / year Rubella: 186,000 reported cases per year. Rubella epidemic in 1964–1965 in the United States resulted in 12.5 million cases. Since vaccine introduction Measles: 99% reduction in measles Mumps: 99% reduction in disease incidence, but periodic outbreaks occur. In 2016, there were 5,311 reported cases of mumps. Rubella: ~11 reported cases per year (2005–2011)	1st dose: 12–15 months 2nd dose: 4–6 years	Low-grade fever, non-contagious measles-like rash, fever (>103°F), short-lived arthritis or joint inflammation Rare: short-lived decrease in number of platelets circulating in the blood, seizures associated with fever	Two doses are 97% effective against measles, 97% effective against rubella, and 88% effective against mumps.

Vaccine	Disease	Schedule	Possible side effects	Effectiveness
Varicella zoster Live attenuated virus vaccine	Varicella zoster virus (chickenpox) Chickenpox causes a blister-like rash, itching, tiredness, and fever. Chickenpox can be very serious in people with weakened immune systems, infants, and adults.	Before vaccine introduction 4 million cases per year and 1 or 2 deaths among children each week Since vaccine introduction 97% reduction in the number of varicella cases	1st dose: 12–15 months 2nd dose: 4–6 years	Pain, redness, swelling, or soreness at the injection site; low-grade fever. Fever can occur within 42 days of vaccination. Rash with fewer than 10 blisters around injection site or other body parts (3%)	Completion of 2-dose vaccine series 98% effective at preventing chickenpox
Hepatitis A Inactivated virus vaccine	Hepatitis A virus Causes mild to severe liver disease. Symptoms include fever, stomach pain, jaundice (yellowing of the skin), nausea. 15% of cases hospitalized	Before vaccine introduction 30,000–60,000 reported cases per year Since vaccine introduction ~1,600–2,500 reported cases per year	2-dose series between 12 and 23 months; separate the 2 doses by 6–18 months	Pain, redness, and tenderness at the injection site, mild fever, feeling "out of sorts," fatigue	68% reduction in hepatitis A hospitalizations since vaccine introduction

(continued)

Vaccine	Vaccine-Preventable Disease	Brief History	Current Routine Schedule (United States)	Reported Adverse Events[a,b]	Vaccine Effectiveness
Meningococcal conjugate ACWY (MCV4) Meningococcal B (MenB) MCV4: conjugate protein vaccine MenB: recombinant vaccine	*Neisseria meningitides* Bacteria that can cause serious bloodstream infections and meningitis. Fatality rate for severe infection is 10%	Approximately 800–1,500 cases of meningococcal disease occur annually in the United States. Serogroups B, C, and Y cause most infections in the United States. Serogroup B is associated with recent outbreaks on college campuses and now causes a significant proportion of the cases among infants/young children, adolescents, and young adults.	MCV4 1st dose: 11–12 years 2nd dose: 16 years 1- to 4-dose series[c] for infants, young children with certain medical conditions Men B vaccines licensed in 2014 and 2015 2 doses 1 or 6 months apart at age 16–18 years (grade B recommendation) 2- or 3-dose series[c] for adolescents age 10 years or older with certain medical conditions	Pain or tenderness at the injection site, fever (100–103°F), headache Muscle and joint pain also reported with MenB	MCV4 effectiveness 80–85% within 3 years of vaccination

diphtheria-acellular pertussis (Tdap) Adolescent/adult formulation of DTaP Protein subunit vaccine	pertussis (see DTaP entry). history.	dose between 11 and 12 years	and swelling at the injection site; low-grade fever; headache; body aches or muscle weakness; fatigue	protects ~7 out of 10 adolescents against pertussis. However, protection fades over time; ~3 to 4 out of 10 people are fully protected 4 years after receiving the vaccine.
Human papillomavirus (HPV9) Recombinant vaccine	Human papillomavirus HPV is the most common sexually transmitted infection, affecting 80% of all men and women during their lifetime. The majority of new infections occur in 15- to 24-year-olds. Some types of the virus can cause cancers of the anus, cervix, oropharynx, penis, rectum, vagina, and vulva, as well as genital warts. Vaccine protects against 9 HPV types associated with ~85% of cervical cancers.	2-dose schedule: 0, 6–12 months for adolescents aged 11 or 12 years 3-dose schedule for adolescents who receive first HPV dose at age 15 years or older: 0, 1–2, and 6 months	Pain, redness, or swelling at the injection site; slight fever Rare: fainting	Each year in the United States, HPV causes 30,700 cancers in men and women and >300,000 new cases of genital warts. Approximately 70% reduction in prevalence of cancer-causing serotypes observed since vaccine introduction. HPV9 has an estimated potential to prevent 90% of anogenital cancers caused by HPV.

[a]Most commonly reported adverse events: These reported events all self-resolve.

[b]Severe allergic reaction can occur after administration of any vaccine due to allergy to a vaccine component but is very rare (<1 in 1 million doses). Severe allergic reaction to a previous dose or vaccine component is a contraindication to all vaccines. Moderate or severe acute illness with or without fever is a precaution for all vaccines.

[c]Number of doses depends on vaccine brand.

Schedules and Overviews for Common Adult Vaccines

Vaccine	Vaccine-Preventable Disease	Brief History	Current Schedule and Coverage	Reported adverse events[a,b]	Effectiveness
Influenza	See child/adolescent table.	See child/adolescent table.	1 dose annually for ages 19 years or older	See child/adolescent table.	
Tetanus–diphtheria (Td) Tetanus–diphtheria–acellular pertussis (Tdap)	See child/adolescent table.	See child/adolescent table.	All adults age 19 years or older should receive a tetanus booster (Td) every 10 years. Tdap should be substituted for one Td booster if no prior history of Tdap. Pregnant women: 1 Tdap dose during late second or early third trimester during each pregnancy.	See child/adolescent table.	
Measles, mumps, and rubella (MMR)	See child/adolescent table.	See child/adolescent table.	1 or 2 doses depending on indication for ages 19–59 years who have not been previously vaccinated	See child/adolescent table.	
Varicella (VAR)	See child/adolescent table.	See child/adolescent table.	2 doses for ages 19 years or older with no history of chickenpox and who have not been previously vaccinated	See child/adolescent table.	

Vaccine	Description	Notes	Schedule	Side effects	Benefits
Herpes zoster Live, attenuated virus vaccine	Shingles: recurrence of varicella virus infection that causes a painful rash on one region of the body, often the face or torso	There are an estimated 1 million cases of shingles each year in the U.S.	1 dose for ages 60 years or older	Common: redness, pain, swelling, or itching at the injection site; fever (101°F or higher); headache	Reduces risk of developing shingles by 51% and postherpetic neuralgia (PHN) by 67% in adults age 60 years or older
Human papillomavirus (HPV9)	See child/adolescent table.		3 doses for females ages 19–26 years who have not been previously vaccinated 3 doses for males ages 19–21 years who have not been previously vaccinated 3 doses for males ages 22–26 years with additional medical conditions or other indications	See child/adolescent table.	See child/adolescent table.
Pneumococcal conjugate (PCV13) Pneumococcal polysaccharide vaccine (PPS23)	See child/adolescent table (PCV13). PPS23 protects against 23 types of *Streptococcus pneumoniae*	See child/adolescent table (PCV13).	See child/adolescent table.	Common: redness or pain at the injection site Rare: fever, muscle aches, severe local reactions	See child/adolescent table.

(continued)

Vaccine	Vaccine-Preventable Disease	Brief History	Current Schedule and Coverage	Reported Adverse Events[a,b]	Effectiveness
Hepatitis A	See child/adolescent table.		2 or 3 doses for ages 19 years or older who have not been previously vaccinated and who have certain medical conditions or other indications	See child/adolescent table.	See child/adolescent table.
Hepatitis B	See child/adolescent table.		3 doses for ages 19 years or older who have not been previously vaccinated or who have not responded to a first vaccine series		See child/adolescent table.
Meningococcal conjugate ACWY	See child/adolescent table.		1 or more doses for ages 19 years or older who have certain medical conditions		See child/adolescent table.
Meningococcal group B (MenB)			2 or 3 doses for ages 19 years or older who have not been previously vaccinated and who have certain medical conditions		

[a]Most commonly reported adverse events: These reported events all self-resolve.

[b]Severe allergic reaction can occur after administration of any vaccine due to allergy to a vaccine component but is very rare (<1 in 1 million doses). Severe allergic reaction to a previous dose or vaccine component is a contraindication to all vaccines. Moderate or severe acute illness with or without fever is a precaution for all vaccines.

SELECTED BIBLIOGRAPHY

General/Vaccinology

Centers for Disease Control and Prevention. *Epidemiology and Prevention of Vaccine Preventable Diseases*. Hamborsky J, Kroger A, Wolfe S, eds. 13th ed. Washington, DC: Public Health Foundation; 2015.

World Health Organization. Global Vaccine Action Plan. 2011; http://www.who.int/immunization/global_vaccine_action_plan/en/.

State of the National Vaccine Plan. 2014; https://www.hhs.gov/nvpo/national-vaccine-plan/state-of-national-vaccine-plan-annual-report-2014/index.html.

Plotkin S, Orenstein WA, Offit PA, eds. *Vaccines*. 6th ed. London: Elsevier/Saunders; 2013.

American Academy of Pediatrics. In: Kimberlin DW, Brady MT, Jackson MA, Long SS, eds. *Red Book: 2015 Report of the Committee on Infectious Diseases*. 30th ed. Elk Grove Village, IL: American Academy of Pediatrics; 2015.

Moser CA, Offit P. *Vaccines and Your Child: Separating Fact from Fiction*. New York, NY: Columbia University Press; 2011.

Keith LS, Jones DE, Chou CH. Aluminum toxicokinetics regarding infant diet and vaccinations. *Vaccine*. 2002;20(Suppl 3):S13–S17.

Shirodkar S, Hutchinson RL, Perry DL, White JL, Hem SL. Aluminum compounds used as adjuvants in vaccines. *Pharm Res*. 1990;7(12):1282–1288.

Chapter 2: A Brief History of Vaccines

History of Vaccines Project. https://www.historyofvaccines.org/content/about.

Allen A. *Vaccine: The Controversial Story of Medicine's Greatest Lifesaver.*
New York, NY: Norton; 2007.

Offit P. *Vaccinated: One Man's Question to Defeat the World's Deadliest
Diseases.* New York, NY: Smithsonian Books (HarperCollins); 2007.

Victorian Imperialism: Texts and Contexts. In The Norton Anthology of
English Literature: Norton Topics Online. https://www.wwnorton.
com/college/english/nael/victorian/topic_4/civilizing.htm
(accessed February 4, 2017).

Pearson-Patel J. A brief history of vaccines in colonial Africa.
ActiveHistory.ca. http://activehistory.ca/2015/04/a-brief-history-
of-vaccines-in-colonial-africa (accessed February 4, 2017)

Chapter 3: Vaccine Development

Ball R, Horne D, Izurieta H, Sutherland A, Walderhaug M, Hsu
H. Statistical, epidemiological, and risk-assessment approaches to
evaluating safety of vaccines throughout the life cycle at the Food
and Drug Administration. *Pediatrics.* 2011;127(Suppl 1):S31–S38.

Barocchi MA, Black S, Rappuoli R. Multicriteria decision analysis and
core values for enhancing vaccine-related decision-making. *Sci
Transl Med.* 2016;8(345):345ps314.

Eskola J, Kilpi T. Public–private collaboration in vaccine research.
Lancet. 2011;378(9789):385–386.

Hyde TB, Dentz H, Wang SA, et al. The impact of new vaccine
introduction on immunization and health systems: A review of the
published literature. *Vaccine.* 2012;30(45):6347–6358.

Marshall V, Baylor NW. Food and Drug Administration regulation and
evaluation of vaccines. *Pediatrics.* 2011;127(Suppl 1):S23–S30.

Rappuoli R, Black S, Lambert PH. Vaccine discovery and translation of
new vaccine technology. *Lancet.* 2011;378(9788):360–368.

Smith J, Lipsitch M, Almond JW. Vaccine production, distribution,
access, and uptake. *Lancet.* 2011;378(9789):428–438.

Garçon N, Stern PL, Cunningham AL, Stanberry LR. *Understanding
Modern Vaccines: Perspectives in Vaccinology.* New York,
NY: Elsevier; 2011.

Chapter 4: Vaccine Financing and Distribution

Lindley MC, Shen AK, Orenstein WA, Rodewald LE, Birkhead
GS. Financing the delivery of vaccines to children and
adolescents: Challenges to the current system. *Pediatrics.*
2009;124(Suppl 5):S548–S557.

Whitney CG, Zhou F, Singleton J, et al. Benefits from immunization
during Vaccines for Children era—United States, 1994–2013.
MMWR. August 25, 2014;63(16).

Immunization Financing Options. Global Alliance for Vaccines and
Immunization (GAVI). http://www.who.int/immunization/
programmes_systems/financing/analyses/00_briefcase_En.pdf

Chapter 5: Vaccine Safety

Adverse Effects of Vaccines: Evidence and Causality. Washington, DC: The
National Academies Press; 2012.

Immunization Safety Review: Vaccines and Autism. Washington, DC: The
National Academies Press; 2004.

Cook KM, Evans G. The National Vaccine Injury Compensation
Program. *Pediatrics*. 2011;127(Suppl 1):S74–S77.

U.S. Court of Federal Claims Decision in Omnibus Autism Proceeding.
http://www.uscfc.uscourts.gov/omnibus-autism-proceeding.

Kolata G. *Flu: The Story of the Great Influenza Pandemic of 1918 and the
Search for the Virus that Caused It*. New York, NY: Farrar, Strauss, &
Giroux; 1999.

Peer-Reviewed, Published Scientific Articles Related to Vaccines and Autism

DeStefano F, Price CS, Weintraub ES. Increasing exposure to antibody-
stimulating proteins and polysaccharides in vaccines is not
associated with risk of autism. *J Pediatr*. 2013;163(2):561–567.

Farrington CP, Miller E, Taylor B. MMR and autism: Further evidence
against a causal association. *Vaccine*. 2001;19(27):3632–3635.

Fombonne E, Chakrabarti S. No evidence for a new variant of measles–
mumps–rubella-induced autism. *Pediatrics*. 2001;108(4):E58.

Klein NP, Fireman B, Yih WK, et al. Measles–mumps–rubella–varicella
combination vaccine and the risk of febrile seizures. *Pediatrics*.
2010;126(1):e1–8.

Klein NP, Lewis E, Baxter R, et al. Measles-containing vaccines
and febrile seizures in children age 4 to 6 years. *Pediatrics*.
2012;129(5):809–814.

Nelson KB, Bauman ML. Thimerosal and autism? *Pediatrics*.
2003;111(3):674–679.

Peltola H, Patja A, Leinikki P, Valle M, Davidkin I, Paunio M. No
evidence for measles, mumps, and rubella vaccine-associated
inflammatory bowel disease or autism in a 14-year prospective
study. *Lancet*. 1998;351(9112):1327–1328.

Pichichero ME, Gentile A, Giglio N, et al. Mercury levels in newborns
    and infants after receipt of thimerosal-containing vaccines.
    Pediatrics. 2008;121(2):e208–214.

Taylor B, Miller E, Farrington CP, et al. Autism and measles, mumps,
    and rubella vaccine: No epidemiological evidence for a causal
    association. *Lancet.* 1999;353(9169):2026–2029.

Black C, Kaye JA, Jick H. Relation of childhood gastrointestinal disorders
    to autism: Nested case–control study using data from the UK General
    Practice Research Database. *BMJ.* 2002;325(7361):419–421.

DeStefano F, Bhasin TK, Thompson WW, Yeargin-Allsopp M, Boyle
    C. Age at first measles–mumps–rubella vaccination in children with
    autism and school-matched control subjects: A population-based
    study in metropolitan Atlanta. *Pediatrics.* 2004;113(2):259–266.

Fombonne E, Zakarian R, Bennett A, Meng L, McLean-Heywood
    D. Pervasive developmental disorders in Montreal, Quebec,
    Canada: Prevalence and links with immunizations. *Pediatrics.*
    2006;118(1):e139–150.

Hornig M, Briese T, Buie T, et al. Lack of association between measles
    virus vaccine and autism with enteropathy: A case–control study.
    PLoS One. 2008;3(9):e3140.

Hviid A, Stellfeld M, Wohlfahrt J, Melbye M. Association
    between thimerosal-containing vaccine and autism. *JAMA.*
    2003;290(13):1763–1766.

Madsen KM, Hviid A, Vestergaard M, et al. A population-based study
    of measles, mumps, and rubella vaccination and autism. *N Engl J
    Med.* 2002;347(19):1477–1482.

Makela A, Nuorti JP, Peltola H. Neurologic disorders after measles–
    mumps–rubella vaccination. *Pediatrics.* 2002;110(5):957–963.

Mrozek-Budzyn D, Kieltyka A, Majewska R. Lack of association
    between measles–mumps–rubella vaccination and autism
    in children: A case–control study. *Pediatr Infect Dis J.*
    2010;29(5):397–400.

Taylor B, Miller E, Lingam R, Andrews N, Simmons A, Stowe
    J. Measles, mumps, and rubella vaccination and bowel problems
    or developmental regression in children with autism: Population
    study. *BMJ.* 2002;324(7334):393–396.

Heron J, Golding J, Team AS. Thimerosal exposure in infants and
    developmental disorders: A prospective cohort study in the
    United Kingdom does not support a causal association. *Pediatrics.*
    2004;114(3):577–583.

Price CS, Thompson WW, Goodson B, et al. Prenatal and infant exposure to thimerosal from vaccines and immunoglobulins and risk of autism. *Pediatrics.* 2010;126(4):656–664.

Thompson WW, Price C, Goodson B, et al. Early thimerosal exposure and neuropsychological outcomes at 7 to 10 years. *N Engl J Med.* 2007;357(13):1281–1292.

Chapter 6: The Vaccine Schedule

Ahmed F, Temte JL, Campos-Outcalt D, Schunemann HJ, Group AEBRW. Methods for developing evidence-based recommendations by the Advisory Committee on Immunization Practices (ACIP) of the U.S. Centers for Disease Control and Prevention (CDC). *Vaccine.* 2011;29(49):9171–9176.

Duclos P, Durrheim DN, Reingold AL, Bhutta ZA, Vannice K, Rees H. Developing evidence-based immunization recommendations and GRADE. *Vaccine.* 2012;31(1):12–19.

Hinman AR, Orenstein WA, Schuchat A; Centers for Disease Control and Prevention. Vaccine-preventable diseases, immunizations, and MMWR—1961–2011. *MMWR Suppl.* 2011;60(4):49–57.

Smith JC. The structure, role, and procedures of the U.S. Advisory Committee on Immunization Practices (ACIP). *Vaccine.* 2010;28(Suppl 1):A68–A75.

Smith JC, Hinman AR, Pickering LK. History and evolution of the Advisory Committee on Immunization Practices—United States, 1964–2014. *MMWR Morb Mortal Wkly Rep.* 2014;63(42):955–958.

Smith JC, Snider DE, Pickering LK; Advisory Committee on Immunization Practices. Immunization policy development in the United States: The role of the Advisory Committee on Immunization Practices. *Ann Intern Med.* 2009;150(1):45–49.

Walton LR, Orenstein WA, Pickering LK. The history of the United States Advisory Committee on Immunization Practices (ACIP). *Vaccine.* 2015;33(3):405–414.

Dolen V, Talkington K, Bhatt A, Rodewald L. Structures, roles, and procedures of state advisory committees on immunization. *J Public Health Manag Pract.* 2013;19(6):582–588.

Strategic Advisory Group of Experts (SAGE) Terms of Reference. http://www.who.int/immunization/sage/Full_SAGE_TORs.pdf

Shen AK, Spinner JR, Salmon D, et al. Strengthening the U.S. vaccine and immunization enterprise: The role of the National Vaccine Advisory Committee. *Public Health Reports.* ; 2011;126.

Chapter 7: Laws and Standard Practices for Vaccine Administration

Alexander K, Lacy TA, Myers AL, Lantos JD. Should pediatric practices have policies to not care for children with vaccine-hesitant parents? *Pediatrics.* 2016;138(4).

Caplan AL, Hoke D, Diamond NJ, Karshenboyem V. Free to choose but liable for the consequences: Should non-vaccinators be penalized for the harm they do? *J Law Med Ethics.* 2012;40(3):606–611.

Cha SH. The history of vaccination and current vaccination policies in Korea. *Clin Exp Vaccine Res.* 2012;1(1):3–8.

Reiss DR. Compensating the victims of failure to vaccinate: What are the options? *Cornell J Law Public Policy.* 2014;23(3):595–633.

Bushak L. A brief history of vaccines: From medieval Chinese "varioloation" to modern vaccination. http://www.medicaldaily.com/history-vaccines-variolation-378738.

Bryson M, Duclos P, Jolly A, Bryson J. A systematic review of national immunization policy making processes. *Vaccine.* 2010;28(Suppl 1): A6–A12.

Omer SB, Enger KS, Moulton LH, Halsey NA, Stokley S, Salmon DA. Geographic clustering of nonmedical exemptions to school immunization requirements and associations with geographic clustering of pertussis. *Am J Epidemiol.* 2008;168(12):1389–1396.

Omer SB, Pan WK, Halsey NA, et al. Nonmedical exemptions to school immunization requirements: Secular trends and association of state policies with pertussis incidence. *JAMA.* 2006;296(14):1757–1763.

Chapter 8: Vaccine Hesitancy

Assessing the state of vaccine confidence in the United States: Recommendations from the National Vaccine Advisory Committee: Approved by the National Vaccine Advisory Committee on June 9, 2015 [corrected]. *Public Health Rep.* 2015;130(6):573–595.

Edwards KM, Hackell JM; Committee on Infectious Diseases and the Committee on Ambulatory Pediatrics. Countering vaccine hesitancy. *Pediatrics.* 2016;138(3).

Glanz JM, Newcomer SR, Narwaney KJ, et al. A population-based cohort study of undervaccination in 8 managed care organizations across the United States. *JAMA Pediatr.* 2013;167(3):274–281.

Shim E, Grefenstette JJ, Albert SM, Cakouros BE, Burke DS. A game dynamic model for vaccine skeptics and vaccine believers: Measles as an example. *J Theor Biol.* 2012;295:194–203.

Betsch C, Brewer NT, Brocard P, et al. Opportunities and challenges of Web 2.0 for vaccination decisions. *Vaccine.* 2012;30(25):3727–3733.

Jarrett C, Wilson R, O'Leary M, Eckersberger E, Larson HJ. Strategies for addressing vaccine hesitancy—A systematic review. *Vaccine.* 2015;33(34):4180–4190.

Larson HJ, Jarrett C, Eckersberger E, Smith DM, Paterson P. Understanding vaccine hesitancy around vaccines and vaccination from a global perspective: A systematic review of published literature, 2007–2012. *Vaccine.* 2014;32(19):2150–2159.

Moser CA, Reiss D, Schwartz RL. Funding the costs of disease outbreaks caused by non-vaccination. *J Law Med Ethics.* 2015;43(3):633–647.

Phadke VK, Bednarczyk RA, Salmon DA, Omer SB. Association between vaccine refusal and vaccine-preventable diseases in the United States: A review of measles and pertussis. *JAMA.* 2016;315(11):1149–1158.

Rosselli R, Martini M, Bragazzi NL. The old and the new: Vaccine hesitancy in the era of the Web 2.0. Challenges and opportunities. *J Prev Med Hyg.* 2016;57(1):E47–E50.

Smith MJ. Promoting vaccine confidence. *Infect Dis Clin North Am.* 2015;29(4):759–769.

Chapter 9: On the Horizon

Berlanda Scorza F, Tsvetnitsky V, Donnelly JJ. Universal influenza vaccines: Shifting to better vaccines. *Vaccine.* 2016;34(26):2926–2933.

Giersing BK, Modjarrad K, Kaslow DC, Okwo-Bele JM, Moorthy VS. The 2016 Vaccine Development Pipeline: A special issue from the World Health Organization Product Development for Vaccine Advisory Committee (PDVAC). *Vaccine.* 2016;34(26):2863–2864.

Higgins D, Trujillo C, Keech C. Advances in RSV vaccine research and development—A global agenda. *Vaccine.* 2016;34(26):2870–2875.

Holzmann H, Hengel H, Tenbusch M, Doerr HW. Eradication of measles: Remaining challenges. *Med Microbiol Immunol.* 2016;205(3):201–208.

Loharikar A, Dumolard L, Chu S, Hyde T, Goodman T, Mantel C. Status of new vaccine introduction—Worldwide, September 2016. *MMWR Morb Mortal Wkly Rep.* 2016;65(41):1136–1140.

Marston HD, Lurie N, Borio LL, Fauci AS. Considerations for developing a Zika virus vaccine. *N Engl J Med.* 2016;375(13):1209–1212.

Melero I, Gaudernack G, Gerritsen W, et al. Therapeutic vaccines for cancer: An overview of clinical trials. *Nat Rev Clin Oncol.* 2014;11(9):509–524.

O'Connor P, Jankovic D, Muscat M, et al. Measles and rubella elimination in the WHO region for Europe: Progress and challenges. *Clin Microbiol Infect.* 2017 doi: 10.1016/j.cmi.2017.01.003. [Epub ahead of print]

Rottingen JA, Gouglas D, Feinberg M, et al. New vaccines against epidemic infectious diseases. *N Engl J Med.* 2017;376(7):610–613.

Soema PC, Kompier R, Amorij JP, Kersten GF. Current and next generation influenza vaccines: Formulation and production strategies. *Eur J Pharm Biopharm.* 2015;94:251–263.

Toole MJ. So close: Remaining challenges to eradicating polio. *BMC Med.* 2016;14:43.

Alchin DR. HIV vaccine development: An exploratory review of the trials and tribulations. *Immunol Res.* 2014;60(1):35–37.

van der Burg SH, Arens R, Ossendorp F, van Hall T, Melief CJ. Vaccines for established cancer: Overcoming the challenges posed by immune evasion. *Nat Rev Cancer.* 2016;16(4):219–233.

INDEX

Page numbers followed by *f* indicate figures; *t* indicate tables.

Printed in the USA/Agawam, MA
October 27, 2017

661352.006